A History of

Brentry

House, Reformatory, Colony and Hospital

By Peter K Carpenter

F.R.C.Psych.

2002

Published 2002 by

Friends of Glenside Hospital Museum
    UWE Glenside Campus
    Stapleton
    Bristol
    BS16 1DD

Registered Charity No: 1042422

Further copies obtainable from:

    Friends of Glenside Hospital Museum price £10 (+ £2 P&P in UK)

ISBN 0-9542458-1-4

Acknowledgements

This account of Brentry could not have occurred without the support of many people. It started when I became worried about the loss of the records of the local hospitals and was enabled by Alison Filer to collect what was still to be found. Then many managers tolerated my disappearance into the cellars and my commandeering of an empty room to store things. Out of this came a collection that went to the Bristol Record Office whose staff then accepted the further depositions and odd requests with magnanimity.

I am also grateful to all the staff who worked in Phoenix NHS Trust who realised my interest and sent me further documents and photographs as they were found.

In addition a large number of people have helped me with accounts of the past and with commenting on drafts of the book. Amongst these can be included Dr Lumsden-Walker, Jim Telling, Jim Phillips, Ann Skeuse, Mavis Beames, Brendan Sheridan, Dr John Harrison, Dr Sylvia Carpenter, Alan Carpenter and Liz Boomer.

Other people have helped with encouragement and advice on preparing the text. This book, though would not have been printed without the financial interest and support of Countryside Properties.

Almost all of the primary sources used for researching this book have been deposited in Bristol Record Office or Bristol Central Reference Library.

Unless stated otherwise the primary records used including the annual reports and printed minutes of the Management Board as well as of the Hospital Management Committee minutes (*HMC*) are deposited in the Bristol Record Office (*BRO*).

However, some of the older records are deposited in Gloucestershire Record Office (*GLRO*) and the Public Record Office (*PRO*) – this is noted where appropriate.

I have endeavoured to make this history as accurate as possible and both I and the Friends of Glenside Hospital Museum would welcome to be told of any errors. I apologise in advance if anyone feels that they are been portrayed in an unfair light.

The Glenside Hospital Museum houses memorabilia of all the old long stay hospitals of Bristol, including Brentry and the Stoke Park Group. It therefore seemed fitting to ask them to agree to publish this book. At present it is routinely open on Wednesday and Saturday mornings, in the old chapel on the University of West of England Glenside Campus.

Peter Carpenter
Kingswood CLDT
Hanham Road,
Bristol BS15 8PQ

1 July 2002

Contents

Illustrations

Introduction

People travelling between Bristol and Cribbs Causeway rarely notice the only large house that they will pass on Passage Road at the top of the hill at Brentry. The transition of the road from a 30 mile an hour zone to a dual carriageway takes all their attention and the low formal house in Bath Stone that is set back above the road to take advantage of the view misses their gaze. But this 'villa' now celebrates its 200th anniversary and is about to start another phase in its life, as the core of a residential development.

This will be the sixth life of the estate. It was first a field and wood, though some say that the name indicates that vines were grown on the slopes. A new life started in 1802 when William Payne had Humphrey and John Repton build Brentry Villa for him and his family and design a surrounding garden. It does not seem to have been a formal garden but a rural romantic idyll of lawns, trees and grotto, framing the view towards Henbury and the Severn Estuary. William soon sold the house to John Cave, an important figure in the commerce and politics of Bristol, who enlarged the estate and house to produce the columned veranda and conservatory that we see now. His son further enlarged it, but soon lost interest in the estate and rented it out before selling it. The Miller's were the final family to own the estate, but the house and estate appears to have become unloved and was abandoned, being sold for less than half the price it was bought for.

At the start of this century, the estate started its third life as a Reformatory for inebriates. It was the first and last inebriate Reformatory in England, and as such launched the career of the Rev. Harold Burden, and its rise and fall as a reformatory marks the tempo of this little known chapter in social reform. It was funded by persuading local councils to purchase beds and thereby a seat on the managing committee and became a hybrid run by a consortium of distant councils and a group of philanthropists. As a Reformatory it incarcerated men and women who would otherwise have been sent to prison. Many of them may well have preferred the shorter prison sentence and several mutinied or escaped. The magistrates soon felt that the place did not cure inebriates and the system collapsed.

At this time though the Mental Deficiency Act had just been passed, which expected councils to provide colonies for mental defectives. The councils that managed Brentry were pleased to have a place to house mental defectives, and so in 1917 Brentry admitted its first male mental defectives and started the fourth phase of its life, as a colony. It took several years for the institution to change from its old prison or workhouse environment to something that resembled a colony that provided a home for life. Several notable people worked there, but none seem to have been engaged in the debate on compulsory sterilisation that was raging during the 1930s, or in other national debates on care, and Brentry stayed as a quiet backwater.

After the Second World War came the social reforms of the Labour Government and Brentry joined the NHS as Brentry Hospital and thus entered its fifth life. As a hospital it was meant to be therapeutic, but in fact the post war period brought staff and financial shortages, with over-crowded, deteriorating wards, that was not improved until the national care scandals of around 1970 forced the government to invest more in people with a mental handicap. It was then intended to run the hospital down and close it, but this took 30 years. Only now can the site enter its new phase as a residential development, sweeping away most of the signs of its life as an institution, and of the 5000 or so people admitted to it.

What has happened at Brentry though, has been a reflection of many national events. Thus the creation of Brentry Villa reflects national fashions and economic forces. The rise and fall of the Inebriate Reformatory and its transformation to a Mental Deficiency Colony and an NHS Hospital was experienced in many other institutions around the country. Its closure and sale to become a housing estate also mimics what has happened at many sites around the country.

This book will attempt to tell the story of the estate. It has many shortcomings. The first is the lack of skill in its writing style. I will apologise in advance for the dry writing style with its lack of personal detail or fantasy about people's motives. The dryness comes from my background as a scientist and my desire to be accurate rather than a theorist. Secondly there are also many holes in the story because the records of Brentry are very patchy. We learn of the creation of Brentry and its life as a family home only from incidental records such as Repton's description of his works, or newspaper adverts. As a result we have to guess at when various additions were made from maps and plans that may well be inaccurate. It's history as an institution prior to 1948 is documented by the committee minutes but these were designed to always reassure councillors and the public. At this time the records of the inmates are almost non-existent and we know of them mainly from newspaper articles or from when they disturbed the smooth running of the place. The committee records become more sparse as the century progresses, until they almost disappear in the 1980s, but during this time the records of the patients increases as clinical files are kept. These however are bound by rules of confidentiality, so those that are used here are heavily doctored to make them unidentifiable. All of the older records, though are now being destroyed so the people will disappear apart from their names in the admission and discharge books. The records that never survived though, are those of the middle staff – the staff who kept the place open and cared for the inmates, patients and resident service users. Few personnel records were kept and none have survived, so the heroes who were prepared to work the long hours and low pay now only survive in the memories of past residents and staff. This is the great unknown history of Brentry and of all other institutions – the history of the ordinary staff.

This book will focus on life in Brentry. In doing so it omits any extensive reference to the development of community services for 'inebriates', or for people with mental deficiency or with a learning disability. As such it tells only a partial story, but to write a fuller story of people who have been served by Brentry would have taken more time and effort than was available to me.

Whilst this book will try to relate events within Brentry to those outside, it will try to ascribe few motives to the people within Brentry. This is because I am wary of so doing. The vocabulary we use to describe our motives changes with time, just as the language we use to describe our service users changes. To say that the Rev. Burden did things for one reason or another, simply begs the question of 'in whose view'. The motive ascribed by us will change as surely as we change our current vocabularies of motive. In a similar way I have used the language of the times. The people admitted to Brentry as 'mental defectives' were a different group to those more recently admitted as 'service users with learning difficulties'. Some of the mental defectives were of above average intelligence, and the term included people who were inebriates, unmarried women in receipt of public assistance, and children who were prosecuted as juvenile delinquents. To claim that these groups are the same as those admitted today and that the modern terminology should be applied to the people of the past does a disservice to all those involved in portraying history accurately. Therefore this history will use many terms that are now considered insulting and offensive, to describe the people of the past, as these were the terms then in use. The insult is not in the names themselves, but in how you, the reader choose to think of people labelled with the names.

Many of the signs of Brentry's old life are now being built over, just as Repton's original Villa has been almost totally hidden by the extensions made to it. The name of the site is to be changed to Royal Victoria Park, and of the house to Repton Hall. All that will be left may well become the ghosts that are said to live at Brentry.

Baden Powell is said to have ghosts in the basement – not because anyone has seen something but because of the creepy feeling that occurs when working in the basement in the old police cells. The area is damp and mouldy and doors open and shut unbidden, but is the feeling of a ghost just the emotions of the people who work there and the damp of the building? We have no record of a person dying there but the cells might well have been the scene of such an event.

At least one person has seen a ghost in the main house. She is described as a silent lady in a dark dress, dressed in the style of the female reformatory inmates or of the female attendants at that time. She was seen walking through various places in the house, including the entrance hall. Who she is we do not know, as the history of the ordinary staff is one of the great mysteries of Brentry. She though may prove to be one of the few people that people remember in the years to come.

This history must be seen as an incomplete and very inadequate one. For the reasons stated earlier, errors must occur. In the earlier histories I am dependant on written material, much of which was written from a biased point of view or with an eye to publicity. In the more recent history the errors are compounded by the faults and biases of human memory and recall, as well as my recall of the stories of others. Ironically in the destruction of some buildings and renovation of others, we may well be able to acquire more information to add to a new history of Brentry. I hope though that this account fuels many recollections and I would welcome any comments, corrections or personal accounts.

Brentry House

Prior to Brentry House there was little of note on Brentry Hill, apart from its beautiful views and sheltered sweep of fields. Brentry House was built there during a lull in the French Wars for a Bristol merchant named William Payne. Payne was an ironmonger who was prospering. He had become a partner with Thomas Daniel and John Scandrett Harford in an important Iron Merchandising company.[1] Thomas Daniel's main money came from a sugar plantation in Barbados. The Quaker Harford was a very wealthy banker who was one of a family of ironmasters in South Wales who are immortalised in Alexander Cordell's *The Rape of the Fair Country*. Harford had recently bought Blaise Castle and moved there to supervise the building of a new house and romantic garden using the services of a local architect William Patey with the help of the up and coming architect John Nash[2] and his new partner, the garden designer Humphrey Repton.

We do not know if William Payne was also a Quaker. He lived in Bristol[3] but appears to have wanted to emulate his partners. Thomas Daniel lived in Henbury. Harford moved nearby to Blaise Castle in 1795. William Payne first moved out of Bristol to Sea Mills where he leased Riverside House.[4] He then felt he needed to be in a more prestigious place closer to his partners and in 1797[5] purchased a field on Brentry Hill and commissioned Repton to design both a house and garden for him.

Humphrey Repton was the last of the three great landscape gardeners who dominated the English Landscape movement of the eighteenth century. He was born in Suffolk in 1752 and became a country gentleman in a small estate in Norfolk.[6] Poverty forced him to move to Essex and to become a landscape gardener in 1788. He taught himself surveying and studied the gardens of Capability Brown and others as he launched his new career. He was asked to improve the landscapes or houses at over 200 houses in England, including locally Blaise Castle, Dyrham Park, Oldbury Court, Red Fort (now the University of Bristol), Leigh Court, Kingsweston and Ashton Court. For most he produced his famous "Red Books" illustrating the proposed landscapes, but the one for Brentry does not survive.

Humphrey Repton was at the height of his powers. Unfortunately the middle of the French wars meant that few great gardens were being commissioned so much of the work of this time was for

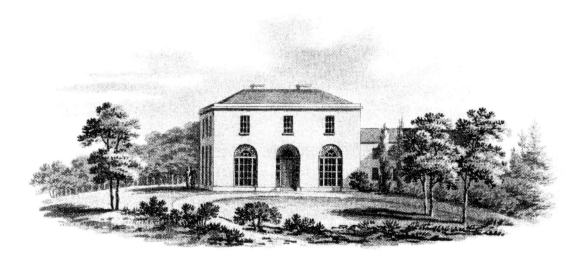

Figure 2.1: 'Villa at Brentry Hill, near Bristol' Reptons drawing of his new house. Notice that the house is square with three windows on each side.

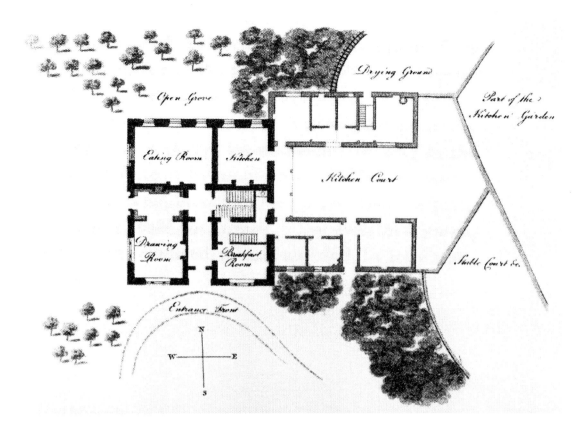

Figure 2.2: Plan of Repton's Brentry Villa

gentlemen who needed modest residences and gardens. He had already worked at Blaise Castle and Kingsweston and would have known the area well. He probably met William Payne during visits to Blaise Castle and may even have been the person who suggested to William Payne that Brentry Hill was an ideal site for a house. The site selected for the house was certainly spectacular at the top of a valley, with glorious views over Henbury and the Severn Estuary combined with a hill flank giving shelter from westerly winds and a plateau behind for the kitchen garden.

Humphrey Repton worked on Brentry and its estate with his son John Repton who had been working as an architect with John Nash. They were sufficiently pleased with the house to exhibit a view and plan of the 'villa' (Figures 2.1 and 2.2) at the Royal Society for Arts in 1802, the year the house was finished.[7] In addition Humphrey Repton was so pleased with the house and its setting that he wrote at length on it.

> A field of a few acres called BRENTRY HILL, near Bristol, commands a most pleasing and extensive view. In the foreground are the rich woods of King's Weston, and Blaize Castle, with the picturesque assemblage of gardens and villas in Henbury and Westbury; beyond which are the Severn and Bristol Channel, and the prospect is bounded by the mountains of South Wales. This view is towards the west, and I have generally observed that the finest prospects in England are all towards this point. Yet this, of all aspects, is the most unpleasant for a house; it was not therefore advisable to give an extended front in this direction, yet it would have been unpardonable not to have taken advantage of so fine a prospect. ...
> Under this restraint perhaps a few houses have been built with more attention to the situation and circumstances of the place, than the villa at Brentry. The eating-room is to the north, with one window towards the prospect, which may be opened or shut out by Venetian blinds at pleasure. The breakfast room is towards the south, and the drawing-room towards the prospect.

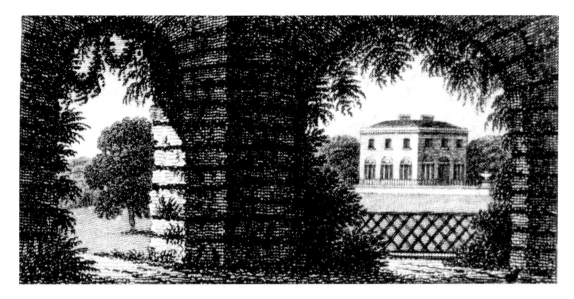

Figure 2.3: 'The GROTTO at BRENTRY HILL, BRISTOL – Seat of Wm Payne Esq[r]

Modern habits have altered the uses of a drawing-room: formerly the best room in the house was opened only a few days in each year, where the guests sat in a formal circle, but now the largest and best room in a gentleman's house is that most frequented and inhabited: it is filled with books, musical instruments, tables of every description, and whatever can contribute to the comfort or amusement of the guests, who form themselves into groups, at different parts of the room; and in winter, by the help of two fire-places, the restraint and formality of the circle is done away.

This has been often happily effected in old houses by laying two rooms together, preserving the fire-places in their original situations, without regard to correspondence in size or place; but two fires not being wanted in summer, a provision is made in this villa to preserve an additional window towards the fine prospect at that season of the year; and the pannel [*sic*], which ornaments the end of the room, may be removed in winter, when the window will be less desirable than a fire-place; thus the same room will preserve, in every season, its advantages of aspects and of views, while its elegance may be retained without increasing the number of rooms for different purposes....

Another circumstance may be mentioned, in which economy has been consulted at this small villa. More rooms are generally required on the chamber than on the ground floor; yet, except the kitchen, there is no part of a house which ought properly to be so lofty as the principal rooms; instead, therefore, of increasing the quantity of offices, by what a witty author calls, "turning the kitchen out of doors for smelling of victuals," this offence is here avoided by the external passage of communication.[8]

One can only hope that the short walk outside to keep the smells away from the principal rooms did not produce cold food.

At this time Repton often used a gothic style but at Brentry, as with many of his smaller villas, he used the Grecian style. How much of this was the work of Humphrey and how much of John is unclear, but there is much in the designs of the lower windows that John would have learnt from John Nash. The fluted semi-circular tympanums had appeared in several other works of John Nash. Dorothy Stroud suggests that they ultimately derive from the venetian windows in Robert Adam's façade for the Royal Society of Arts where Repton exhibited his drawing of Brentry.[9] Nash's first use of the window style was at Llanaeron, in Cardiganshire, built in 1794. Later examples were built whilst John Repton worked for him: Point Pleasant in Surrey, built in 1796-7 and Southgate Grove in Old Southgate, Middlesex, built in 1797.[10] It is said that by the time of

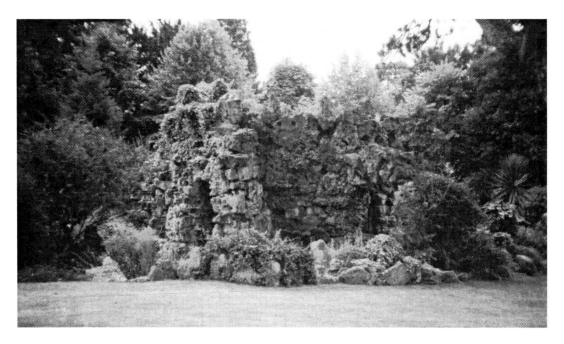

Figure 2.4: The Grotto at Bath Spa Hotel.

Brentry, Nash was "too flashy an architect to produce much in the restrained Neo-classical style."[11] John Repton clearly continued to use the designs he was familiar with from working in Nash's offices.

Humphrey Repton was primarily a landscape gardener and laid out a garden, walks, and a scenic entrance driveway. Unfortunately we know almost nothing of these other than the fact that he possibly built a grotto as he published an illustration of one (Figure 2.3). From the illustration, the grotto appears to have been a rustic structure above ground,[12] more like the grotto in the current garden of the Bath Spa Hotel (Figure 2.4, built after 1836) than the underground eighteenth century grotto at Goldney Hall.[13] The grotto at Brentry was probably linked by a passage to the neighbouring old quarry, (which is now on the edge of Passage Road, and contains the remains of an old electricity substation). A mouldy file from 1932 found in the cellar of the house records a series of passages that were probably found about here,[14] which had been artificially constructed and lined in much the same way as the grotto in Goldney Hall. The plan of the passages shows three entrances but none can be found now so they must have been filled in. These passages gave rise to the legend that there are passages running from the house to the Passage Road quarry, but there is no evidence to show that they ran as far as the house and it would have been unusual for this to have happened.[15]

At this time Charlton Road ran near the house so a line of trees and shrubs was planted to screen the house from the road. The old road can still be traced continuing the straight line of Charlton Road behind the new Hospice, to pass the house along the line of woods. Repton does not illustrate the Stable Block or the workshops, but he must have built the core of the stable building that still exists (Figure 2.5), namely the end closest to the main house which has a classical simplicity to it.[16]

In June 1807, about five years after he commissioned it, William Payne put the estate up for sale and moved back to Bristol.[17] Why he did so is unknown - but like other merchants he may well have been falling on hard times with the Napoleonic wars. Fortunately the sale notice gives a good impression of the estate as it was first built, and suggests that Repton's Breakfast Room had become a Library.

BRINTRY HOUSE
To be sold by auction at the Exchange Coffee Room
on Tuesday 25 August at 1 o'clock....
A most desirable, elegant and modern Mansion HOUSE, newly built with Bath
Stone, the residence of WILLIAM PAYNE Esq., ... commanding most extensive
and picturesque views of the River Severn, the Welch Coast, the village of
Henbury, Blaize Castle, and the adjoining country.
Also the Gardens, inclosed with Brick fruit walls 14 feet high, Melon-ground,
hothouses, shrubberies, coach-houses, stall-stabling for 10 horses, and 65
acres of LAND in a ring fence, surrounding the Mansion House...
The ground floor of the House consists of a dining room 26 feet by 20 feet,
drawing room 27 feet by 19 feet, library 14 feet by 16 feet, hall, Portland stone
staircase, butler's pantry, china pantry, servants' hall, dairy, larder, and excellent
kitchens and other offices.
For Further particulars, and for tickets to view the Premises, which will only be
shewn between the hours of Eleven and One o'clock, apply to Messrs. JOHN &
JEREMIAH OSBORNE, Broad Street, Bristol.[18]

A remodel by the Caves

The house was bought by John Cave. He was a powerful banker in his 50s whose power was
still growing. His father had started the bank of Ames, Cave & Co. and two of his brothers were
partners in the bank. His brother and sister had married the children of William Payne's partner,
the wealthy Thomas Daniel, whose son Thomas joined the bank. John Cave was a director of the
Bristol Dock Company by 1808,[19] and became a founding director of Brunel's Great West
Railway.[20] As a partner of the Phoenix Glass Works Company[21] he also had part ownership of
several ships who traded with the Americas.[22] He became Mayor of Bristol in 1828. He seems to
have spent a lot of money expanding and rebuilding his residence at Brentry to make it
something more appropriate for someone of his status.

Starting in about 1817, he acquired another 150 acres of land surrounding the estate, including
Brentry Farm on Charlton Road. In 1825 he then moved Charlton Road away from the main
house to its present route avoiding the house.[23] A new private drive and gate lodge were built and
the Grotto was presumably demolished at the same time as it would have compromised the new
entrance drive and Grottos were unfashionable by the 1820s.

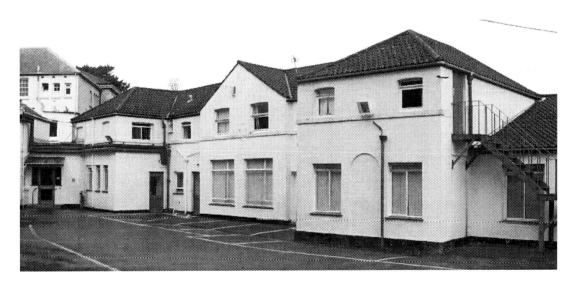

Figure 2.5: What is probably the original Repton Stable Block, in March 2000.

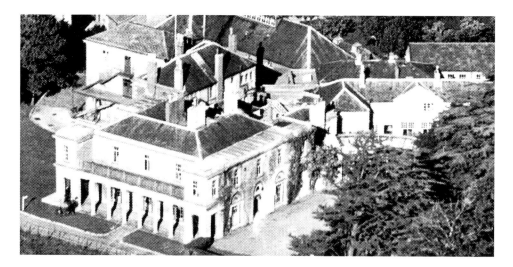

Figure 2.6: Brentry House showing roof of extension made about 1825 and additional storey above old kitchen, added after fire in 1904.

John Cave first enlarged the main house by converting the Kitchen into a library.[24] To do this he rebuilt the north wing of the kitchen court, moving the kitchen into it (illustrated in Figure 4.12). The ceiling height needed by the new kitchen meant that the rooms above needed additional stairs to get to them. In addition he appears to have built a bathroom (which probably had a cold plunge pool) by the kitchen. He probably also extended the Stable Block and outhouses.

After this he appears to have decided he needed a larger house and soon after 1825 radically altered the main house including the two main frontages. He rebuilt the entire wall of the south side of the house, bringing it forward towards the road by about ten feet. In doing so he lengthened the drawing room and library/breakfast room. He left the original site of the front door unchanged, but now recessed with an outside entrance lobby to shelter in. The conservatory was probably built at the same time as moving the wall forward enabled the conservatory to open off the breakfast room and form a continuous line with the front of the house. The entrance frontage was extended with towers at each end, one disguising the join with the conservatory, the other the fact that the west frontage had been extended to four windows. The extension produced a strip of flat roof on the side of the house (Figure 2.6) and made the pitched roof of the main building seem lopsided when viewed from the west, from the main garden. The architect visually disguised this defect in the roof-line by adding the north west tower diagonally onto the corner of the building, and linked the towers into the design by adding a veranda. The finished image was impressive. (Figure 2.11)

The architect for these changes is not known, but it is tempting to assume that it was John or his younger brother George Repton. The curved conservatory recalls the curved conservatory John Nash built at Blaise Castle in 1806 whilst George Repton worked with him, and one feels that whoever rebuilt the entrance front must have had some sympathy or fondness for the designs of John Repton's windows to go to the trouble of rebuilding them and adding another. Nash was in Bristol in 1810-12 building Blaise Hamlet and Harford's Bank but there is no evidence he was in Bristol again or was involved in the alterations at Brentry. Humphrey Repton died in 1818, but two of his sons continued to practice as architects: George Repton emulated his elder brother and worked in John Nash's offices until 1820 when he worked independently until he retired in 1845.[25] John Repton continued to practice as an architect designing houses for several years after the death of his father and worked for a time abroad. The central columned veranda of Brentry is reminiscent of his design for Sheringham Hall, which Humphrey and John designed in 1812.[26]

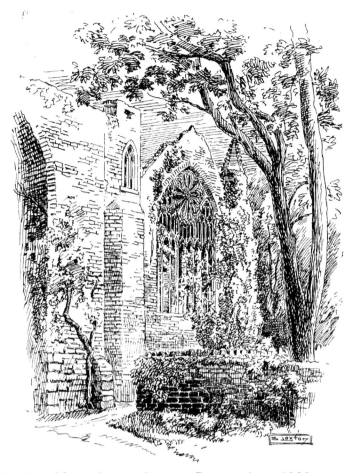

Figure 2.7: 'The Lookout' from the south-west, Drawn about 1900.

John Cave is stated to be responsible also for a folly on the other side of Passage Road. John Latimer writes that in 1822, when the Lord Mayor's Chapel on College Green was extensively repaired, John Cave used the stones of the old west wall and window to build a ruin in Sheepswood. [27] This ruin (Figure 2.7) is marked on Bryant's 1824 Map of Gloucestershire as 'The Lookout' and is still standing behind the houses of Chapel Close. The oddity about this account is that John Cave was not a member of the Bristol Common Council in 1822 as Latimer claims, but he became one in 1824. More importantly, there is no evidence that John Cave ever owned the land that the Lookout is built on. However John's son William lived at the other side of Sheepswood, in Henbury Hill House (opposite the entrance to Blaise Castle) and rented the land adjacent to John Cave's, from Henbury Hill House to Passage Road, the area currently covered by Northover Road, the Ridgeway and the Theological College.[28] Within this is the part of Sheepswood where the Lookout was built.[29] John may have been influential in getting the stones for his son, who would have liked a monument to improve the view from his house. The Lookout would have provided a pleasant break on the walk between the two houses and may have been visible from Brentry as well as Henbury Hill House when the trees were smaller.

John Cave's wife Penelope[30] died before he did, and in 1841, John lived at Brentry House with his daughter Catherine, surrounded by 2 male servants and 5 female servants. His son, William, lived nearby with his wife Mary, and six children. John Cave died in 1842, [31] but William did not move into Brentry House so Catherine may have continued to live there until the estate was advertised for sale in 1847: This advert shows how the estate had changed with John Cave's building work:

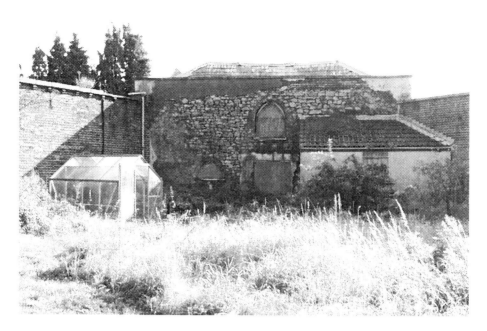

Figure 2.8: the back of Boundary Cottage that faces the garden, showing continuing evidence of the original design as a gothic triangular garden house.

TO BE SOLD BY PRIVATE CONTRACT, THE BRENTRY ESTATE - comprising capital MANSION HOUSE, late the residence of JOHN CAVE Esq.; PLEASURE GROUNDS, PLANTATION, ORCHARD, Two Walled GARDENS, HOT-HOUSES, Etc, FARM-HOUSE and BUILDINGS, COTTAGES and ENTRANCE LODGE, with 212 Acres of productive pastures, Arable and WoodLAND ...

The Mansion House is in perfect order, and replete with every convenience, and contains, on the Ground Floor, large entrance Hall, drawing room 38 feet by 16 feet, dining room 25 feet by 18, and library 18½feet by 16; breakfast room 20 feet by 16 opening into spacious Conservatory facing the Pleasure Ground; bathroom 16 feet by 8; servants hall, butlers pantry, kitchen, water closet and other conveniences. On the first floor are four large best bedrooms, three dressing rooms, a sitting room, and water closet, and six other bedrooms.

The Domestic Offices are most complete and spacious, comprising Store room, Brew house, Dairy, Larder, &c; there are 3 stables, two coach houses, saddle room, laundry, &c detached from the premises, with an abundant supply of both sorts of water.

The Estate is beautifully wooded; and the Orchard and Gardens are well stocked with productive Fruit Trees and contain Hot Forcing and Green Houses...[32]

This description shows that by this time there were more alterations to the estate. In particular the kitchen garden had been split into two gardens. Presumably this was to provide a secluded flower garden by the house. At the same time, one might expect the gothic garden house (Figure 2.8) to have been built into the corner to create the house now extended and known as 'Boundary Cottage' (from the old parish and county boundary stone that that remains). Also from the description the stable block appears to have been extended. Rather oddly these changes are not shown in the 1841 tithe map of the area, which does not show the conservatory or other alterations either. This implies that either all the building works occurred between 1841 and 1847, when there was no clear reason for them, or the map is simplified. It seems much more likely that John Cave extended his house to suit his needs, including a flower garden and garden house as he got older, rather than his son had a flurry of expensive activity and then put the estate

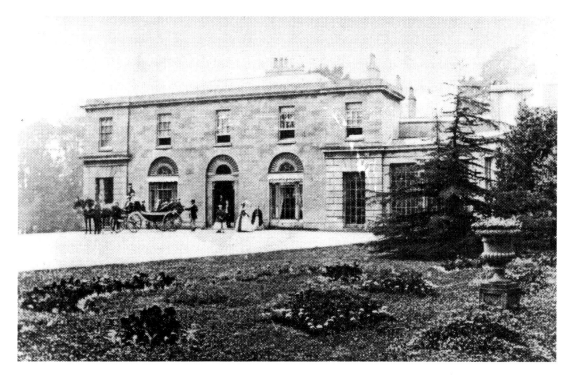

Figure 2.9: Brentry House and family. It is difficult to date this photograph which could be between 1850 and 1870.

up for sale. One odd feature of all the alterations is that there does not seem to have been a great increase in the number of grand bedrooms. This would be in keeping with the needs of John who lived with only his wife and daughter, rather than those of his son who had six children living with him.

After advertising the house for sale, William seems to have changed his mind as the estate was withdrawn from sale. Why he changed his mind is not clear but his first wife died at about this time. In 1850[33] William remarried a young woman, Louisa, who was only three years older than his eldest daughter. He then left Henbury Hill House, which would have been full of memories of his first wife and moved to Brentry where, in 1851, he was living with Louisa, five children and 11 servants. He probably built the three storey extension in order to provide additional bedrooms and nursery space for his young children, as none would have lived there under John Cave. He may also have added the extension and bay window to the Library, so that it obtained a view of the estate. He did not stay long at the house though, as he advertised the house for rent in 1854.[34] This advert shows the increase in bedroom accommodation that had occurred within seven years.

> BRENTRY HOUSE, NEAR HENBURY, TO BE LET, partly Furnished, on a LEASE of five years, a handsome FAMILY MANSION, with a compact and Park-like estate of about 30 acres. … The house has a noble frontage, and consists of Entrance hall, four commodious reception rooms, eight best Bedrooms, four Dressing-rooms, 2 best Water-closets, eight Servants' Bedrooms, Servants' Hall, Kitchens, and Domestic offices, replete with every convenience. and abundantly supplied with both sorts of Water, with two good Coach-houses and Stabling for ten horses; excellent Walled Kitchen Garden, well stocked…

Why he moved after such a short time is a mystery, but he probably found that his new three storey extension was very unsatisfactory as it was built around the kitchen and would have suffered from the cooking smells.

This second attempt to rent out the estate also seems to have failed though William moved elsewhere as the directories record no-one living at the House until 1858 when a Mrs Cave is briefly resident at 'Brentree'.[35] We do not know if this was William's mother or wife. A photograph of the house exists which appears from the costumes and carriage to be of about this date (Figure 2.9). It shows a group of people with their carriage but who these people are is not known.

Life after the Caves

In 1859 Brentry House was occupied by Edward Clark,[36] a lawyer in Bristol, who in 1861[37] was living there with his wife, 7 children, two other relatives, governess and 10 servants. Given the size of his family it is likely that the three storey extension had been built by then to house them. He may have been renting the property from the Caves, but the house and estate was sold in about 1868 for £23,000 to George Miller, an African Merchant and JP for Bristol.[38] Miller's young family grew up there. His son Audley M. Miller[39] later wrote that he was the first Miller to be born at Brentry and recalled living there for 20 years. In 1871 George was living at Brentry with his wife and four young children.[40] The Millers do not appear to have done much to the house, though it has been claimed that it was George Miller who built the three storey extension and garden house. George Miller died in 1881 at the age of 60[41] and was buried in Henbury Churchyard. The first large scale Ordinance Survey map of 1882 helps to set out how far Brentry had changed from Repton's original design (Figure 2.10)

George left the house in trust for his wife Mary and then to his son Thomas on reaching 25 years[42]. The family continued to live at the house until about 1890. At about this time the Millers left the estate as the House was occupied by only two servants at the time of the 1891 census.[43] By 1899 his wife had moved to Cheltenham, and the son Thomas to Cricklade.[44] Mary died in 1919 aged 81 and was buried next to her husband.

The estate was auctioned on the 28 April 1898 but, yet again, the estate proved difficult to sell. It was withdrawn from sale at £13,500[45] - almost half the price George had paid for it thirty years earlier. Why it was so difficult to sell is unclear - it does not appear to have become dilapidated, but the later extensions must have proved very unsatisfactory, spoiling the appearance of the building whilst providing little accommodation of quality. In November 1898 Thomas rented the estate to the Promoters of the Royal Victoria Homes for a term of 3 years[46] before selling it to them on 26 July 1899, effectively allowing them to pay for it in instalments by providing them with the mortgage for the house.

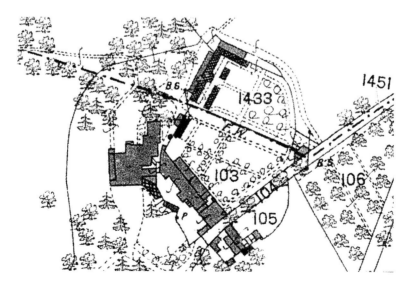

Figure 2.10: Map of Brentry in 1882.

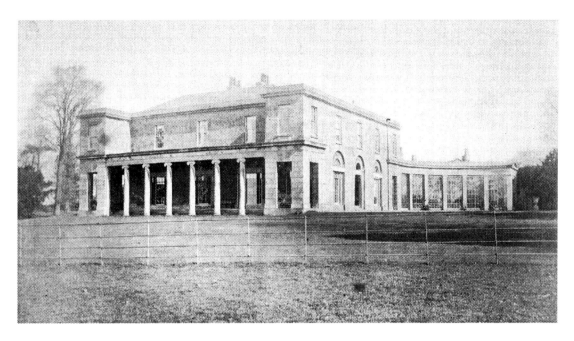

Figure 2.11: Brentry House in about 1900

Notes

[1] For Harford and Daniels see '*A history of banking in Bristol*'

[2] see M Mansbridge: *John Nash - a complete catalogue.* Oxford:Phaidon 1991 page 64f

[3] In Wm Bailey's *The Bristol and Bath Directory.* Bristol 1787 he is an Ironmonger at St Michaels Hill; In 1798 Wm Payne is a Merchant at 59 Queens Square.

[4] BRO: 40775/12.

[5] BRO: P/HTW/OP 1(f) Westbury Poor book - first registers him owning field valued £5-10s in 1797.

[6] For biographical details see George Carter, Patrick Goode and Kedrun Laurie; *Humphrey Repton - landscape gardener 1752-1818.* London: Sainsbury Centre for Visual Arts, 1982.

[7] BRO: P/HTW/OP 1(f) Westbury Poor book shows the value of the field increasing from £5-10s in 1802 to £33 for the 1803 rates onwards.

[8] H Repton: *Observations on the Theory and Practice of Landscape Gardening. Including some remarks on Grecian and Gothic architecture, collected from various manuscripts, in the possession of the different noblemen and gentlemen, for whose use they were originally written; the whole tending to establish fixed principles in the respective arts.* London: J Taylor, 1803 [reprinted Phaidon Press Ltd.]pages 184-6 (incl footnote of final paragraph).

[9] Dorothy Stroud *Humphrey Repton* London 1962. Page 123

[10] M.Mansbridge *John Nash. Op cit.* (note 2)

[11] George Carter *et al: Humphrey Repton..... (op cit* note 6*)* page 79

[12] The site of the grotto is unknown, but from the print is probably by the 'private drive', or under it, close to the quarry bend.

[13] See S. Harding, D Lambert: *Parks and Gardens of Avon.* Bristol: Avon Gardens Trust, 1994

[14] *BRO:* 40686/B/P/6

[15] I am assured that there were passages running from the cellar that have been blocked up in living memory. If so then these are unlikely to have run the distance required, but may have run elsewhere, such as under the conservatory. There is no evidence of passages in the cellars now.

[16] The stable block and outbuildings (mostly now demolished for the Hospice) are in a plan dated 7 Mar 1825 ref: *GLRO:* Q/SRh/1825/A/3

[17] Matthew's *Directory of Bristol* for 1809 shows a Mr William Payne, merchant, living at 33 Park Street.

[18] *Felix Farley's Bristol Journal* 8 August 1807: page1d - also appearing 27 June (2d) to 22 August 1807(2d)

[19] *BRO* 32173/12-13.

[20] John Latimer: *Annals of Bristol in the Nineteenth Century.* Bristol: W & F Morgan, 1887 p189 - he subscribed £17,900.

[21] *BRO* 12143/18,21

[22] G.E.Farr (Ed.) *Record of Bristol Ships 1800 - 1838.* Vol 15 of Bristol Record Society. 1950

[23] Harding and Lambert (*op cit* Note 13) page 64, plan and document dated 7 Mar 1825 ref: *GLRO: Q/SRh/1825/A/3*

[24] The 1825 plan (*GLRO:*Q/SRh/1825/A/3) shows the change in shape of the kitchen block and of the stables, but not the conservatory extension.

[25] For biography of George and John Repton see Appendix in Carter, *et al.: Humphrey Repton. (op cit.)*

[26] See illustrations in D. Stroud: *Humphrey Repton.(op cit.)*

[27] John Latimer: *Annals of Bristol in the Nineteenth Century.* Bristol: W & F Morgan, 1887, p101

[28] BRO: Westbury Tithe map

[29] BRO: Westbury Tithe map and apportionment

[30] C H Cave: *A History of Banking in Bristol.* Bristol:W Crofton Hemmons, 1899; page 224 Penelope was the daughter of Thomas Oliver. William says 1851 born in Bradford Somerset, so John may have lived there in 1805.

[31] HO107/359 f48 (page 12)Deaths J1842 John Cave Clifton, v11p245

[32] *Felix Farleys Bristol Journal* 5 June 1847 page 4f also 22 May page 4c

[33] *Felix Parley's Bristol Journal* 12 October 1850 page5f: on October 8 at Whippingham Church, Isle of Wight by Bishop of Lincoln, William Cave Esq. Of Brentry to Louisa Frances 3rd daughter of late J.H.Butterworth Esq of Clapham Common.

[34] *Bristol Mirror* 9 September 1854 page4c

[35] *Matthews Directory for Bristol 1858*: Westbury on Trym entry

[36] *Matthews Directory of Bristol 1859*; entry for Westbury, and for Attorneys.

[37] 1861 Census RG9/1740/ff46

[38] *Matthew's Bristol Directory with adjacent villages, 1868.* - GLRO:CJ1/C1 states the estate cost him £23,000.

[39] *BRO:* 40686/B/P/6: Caves file of Brentry - letter from A M Miller to Med. Supt -dated 24 Sept 1932 from Heale House, Woodford, Salisbury - he says he is in business at T Paul & Co, 87 Alma Road, Clifton.

[40] 1871 Census RG10/2570/ff49-50

[41] His tombstone in Henbury Churchyard says he died 23 Jan 1881

[42] will dated 19 Nov 1880, George Miller died 1881. this is cited in the conveyance deed of Brentry, dated 26 July 1899, in hands of Bevan Ashford solicitors.

[43] 1891 Census RG12/1989/ff86 - the 74 year old "head servant" says she is "Mistress in charge"

[44] cited in deeds for Brentry held for the Secretary of State by Bevan Ashford Solrs. in Bristol

[45] *Horfield and Bishopston Record and Montpelier and District Free Press.* Saturday 30 April 1898 page 2b

[46] *Horfield and Bishopston Record and Montpelier and District Free Press.* Saturday 26 November 1898 pg 3d

The Move to an Institution.

Brentry moved from being a family home to being an Inebriate Retreat and Reformatory because of the Inebriacy Acts. These were the culmination of a campaign for the treatment of the habitual drunkard which brought together the religious and moral thrust of the Temperance movement and the campaign of medical men and others to see habitual drunkenness as a medical condition needing treatment.

This campaign had lasted for 40 years.[1] The Temperance Movement had been around for longer than this but pressed to close public houses as a cause of social vice and dens of iniquity. Their pressure would continue until several attempts were made at the turn of the century to introduce bills into parliament to restrict public houses. The temperance movement saw drink as a moral problem, with people too weak to resist and creating social problems. It concentrated on the acute problems of alcohol and the acute temptations it produced. It wanted to deal with the drink rather than the habitual drunkard. It campaigners were expected to be tee-totallers.

There were however, other attitudes to alcohol slightly different to those of the temperance movement. These people saw habitual drunkenness as a problem, but did not advocate banning alcohol, and usually were not tee total themselves. For example, in Bristol Mary Carpenter was working with children and young adults, developing local reformatory schools as well as writing about prisons. She repeatedly came into contact with drunks. She advocated not the abolition of drink but "long incarceration and compulsory abstinence from drink" for drunkards who repeatedly came to court.[2]

Medical men also became involved with the habitual drunkard. The pauper insane, who in the past had also been seen as a social and moral problem, had started to be confined in lunatic asylums and were now being studied by the medical staff there. These asylum doctors started collecting statistics on their cases and were soon stating that alcohol abuse was a potent cause of insanity.[3] Doctors such as Thomas Laycock argued that habitual drunkenness was a disease.[4] The Norwich surgeon and asylum proprietor, Dr Donald Dalrymple, became involved in the treatment of drunks and started to advocate Retreats, where a person could shut themselves away to withdraw from using alcohol. He was convinced that 'Retreats' were effective after visiting the voluntary Retreats for the wealthy based in the United States. He became the MP for Bath and in the 1870s pressed for government legislation to create treatment centres for habitual drunkards.

For government though, Habitual Drunkards were a minor social problem when compared with problems such as child labour and education. In addition the compulsory treatment of Habitual Drunkards caused serious questions of principle. As the Home Secretary stated:

> It was wrong in principle: what would amount to an indeterminate sentence should not be subject to the opinion of physicians. It was easy to tell when a lunatic had recovered but how, once the drunkard had become sober, was the physician to know whether or not he was cured? The idea of keeping the "pests of society" in indeterminate confinement was a "new step ... of a most dangerous character."[5]

Dalrymple died prematurely but his campaign was taken up by the British Medical Association [B.M.A.]. In 1874 they set up a committee to continue his work. The campaign continued to meet government opposition: in 1875 the Home Secretary felt that any Bill dealing with such a poorly defined group of persons who included both criminals and lunatics would be difficult to implement and not worth pursuing. As another man remarked, 'man cannot be made sober by Act of Parliament'. However, whilst the government and others resisted any intervention, the message that this was a serious social problem gained more weight. The national consumption of alcohol continued to rise until it peaked in 1876 at 1.3

gallons of spirit and 34.4 gallons of beer per person per year.[6] In addition the number of arrests for drunkenness rose dramatically in London.[7]

The first success of the campaign was an Act of 1879 - *An Act to facilitate the control and care of Habitual Drunkards*.[8] This act described a 'habitual drunkard' as someone who 'cannot be certified as a lunatic, but who due to habitual intemperate drinking is dangerous to him or herself or incapable of managing their affairs'. It allowed that such a person could voluntarily apply to two magistrates to sign away his freedom and be sent to a Licensed Retreat for up to one year, once he had also convinced them he could pay for his time in the Retreat. This Act was to expire after ten years and was clearly seen as experimental. However, even this limited Act was difficult to pass through parliament, and continued to meet resistance in the press, with the *Times* noting that 'we have never yet sanctioned the principle in this country that mere vice should entail the loss of personal liberty'.[9]

The Act was clearly disappointing for the campaigners who wanted to be able to impose compulsory detention. Whilst the B.M.A. created a licensed retreat, called Dalrymple House, it continued to campaign for more legislation. In 1884 the campaigning *Society for the Study and Cure of Inebriety* was formed by a potent group of eminent reformers including doctors and MPs. In 1888[10] the 1879 Act was made permanent and the title 'Habitual Drunkard' changed to 'Inebriate'. This change of name is symbolic of the growing success of the drive to stop seeing the chronic alcoholic as a criminal but to see him as medically ill and worthy of treatment. One of the active MP's in this 1888 Act was the Bristol MP Dr Alfred Carpenter, who openly campaigned for the right of the State to interfere in society to prevent disease.

The campaign for compulsory detention continued, helped by the reports of the Inspector of Retreats, Dr R.W. Branthwaite, who had run Dalrymple House and now reported on the need for more Retreats and the wonderful successes they produced. The campaigners do not seem to have been bothered by the fact that these were mainly voluntary places for a few self selected gentlemen and therefore could not predict the usefulness of a wider provision of compulsory treatment. The campaigners used the same fashionable worries that were also being used with the feeble-minded: there were eugenic concerns that the craving for alcohol could be passed on down families, and that it could corrupt the neighbours. The newspapers publicised the cases of women who had multiple convictions for drunkenness - for example Jane Cakebread who passed 252 convictions by 1893 and Ellen Sweeney who reached 279 convictions in 1895. It was reported that there were 250,000 prison sentences being handed out for drunkenness annually, with a claimed core of 30,000 habitual drunkards.[11] The corruption needed to be stopped before it further weakened the national stock.

The result was the 1898 Inebriates Act[12] which allowed for magistrates to compulsorily send 'Inebriates' to licensed 'Reformatories' for up to 3 years if their council funded such places. These inebriates could be either people convicted of drunkenness four times in a year, or they could be 'criminal inebriates': a person convicted of an imprisonable crime who was drunk at the time of the offence and who the court felt was a 'habitual drunkard'. As one peer remarked in the House of Lords, the Act 'created crime'. It also created a new institution that was closer to a prison than the previous 'voluntary' Retreats, as the people were sent there against their will. It was the first attempt at a medically run prison for people who were unwilling and rational, and was bound to be an interesting experiment.

The Burdens and the Royal Victoria Home

Two of the key people in the creation of the Brentry Inebriate Retreat and Reformatory were the Rev. Harold Nelson Burden and his first wife Katherine.[13] Harold was born in 1860 at Hythe in Kent, the son of a grocer and wine merchant, who died when he was 12. He followed his grandfather as a farmer but was declared bankrupt as a young man and came to work in the East End of London in the slums, where he met his future wife Katherine Garton.

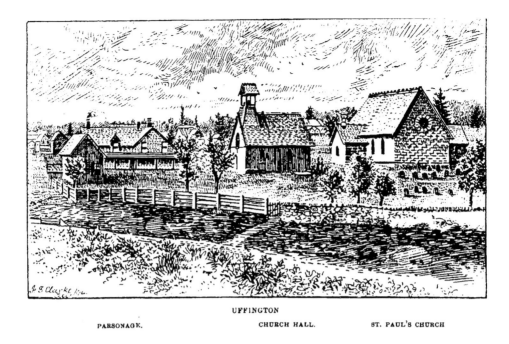

UFFINGTON

PARSONAGE.   CHURCH HALL.   ST. PAUL'S CHURCH

Figure 3.1: The mission in Ontario, Canada that the Burdens built.

'Miss Kate' as she was known, came from a family of snuff manufacturers from Hull and had worked for some time with the well-known reformer, Octavia Hill in the slums. Harold, Kate and others helped set up a Home for young women in the area. In 1888 they heard the Bishop of Algoma, Canada, preach and were inspired to become missionaries in Ontario. Harold was ordained a deacon and the next day they married and left for Canada where they worked for three years building churches and parsonages, (Figure 3.1) only returning because of Harold's ill health and the death of their only two children. Harold probably had chronic heart disease due to childhood rheumatic fever, but this is not definitely known. Certainly he died of inflammation of the heart at the age of almost 70 and had recurrent bouts of illness.

They returned to England where Harold worked in a few posts around London and Cambridge, wrote several books. They arrived in Bristol in 1895 when he took the post of secretary of the Bristol Branch of the Church of England Temperance Society.

From her work Mrs Kate Burden appears as a small energetic, self-effacing lady who had a 'firm faith' and a 'hatred of anything tending to laxity of the moral code'.[14] She probably provided the sense of purpose for her husband but kept out of the limelight as was proper for a Victorian married woman.

The Rev. Harold Burden was an energetic man who eventually developed a national reputation from his management of Inebriate Reformatories and Mental Deficiency Colonies. However there are several confidential writings which later describe him as someone who found it difficult to work with committees. He certainly fell out with many due to his difficulty in surrendering power to others, and this should be borne in mind with several of the events in the early years of the Brentry Institution.[15]

In 1895, when Harold came to Bristol he became clerical secretary of the Church of England Temperance Society. Soon afterwards he also became the honorary secretary of the Police Court and Prison Gate Mission.[16] He now entered into a local project to create a home for women that arose from

> ... the long-cherished desire of the Prison Gate Mission, connected with the CETS [Church of England Temperance Society] to secure a more convenient and commodious shelter.[17]

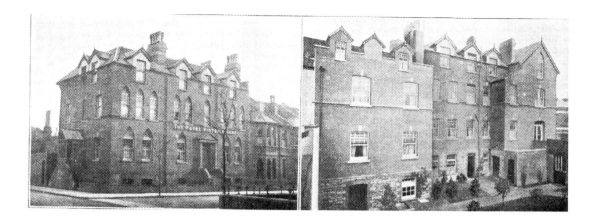

Figure 3.2: The Royal Victoria Home, Horfield.

The basis of this was the lack of an Inebriate Retreat for women in Bristol. There was already a Retreat for men in the area, namely Kingswood Park, started in 1893 and licensed for 20 men.[18] However there was nowhere for the women to go to and the Rev. Burden spearheaded the campaign to create one.

> When the Rev A M [sic] Burden ... became the secretary of the CETS he at once threw himself into a movement so congenial, and for which he was so admirably fitted. ... The funds were collected by the secretary to the CETS from all persons willing to further the particular work, whether such persons belonged to the CETS or not. This eventually led to a difference of opinion as to the precise trusts upon which the property should be held, and necessitated an application to the Charity Commissioners.[19]

The home is elsewhere reported to have started as a home for Inebriates,

> but before it was completed a suggestion came from the Home Office that the work might helpfully also include the care of women convicts ... suitable for the clemency of the Secretary of State. The suggestion was considered a proper one to adopt and a wing was added for their reception.[20]

The resultant hybrid home (Figure 3.2) was called the Women's Shelter Home with Kate as the Lady Superintendent and The Rev. Burden as Chaplain and Secretary[21]. It was immediately afterwards licensed as The Royal Victoria Home (with her Majesty's permission),[22] and was opened to Inebriates as a Retreat in April 1897, with the Burdens joint licensees and living at one end of the property. This became their official Bristol address for 17 years. The building was built by the Prison gates, joined to an older house which was used for the female convicts. Rather bizarrely it also backed on to a Tavern! It was a great success initially, with Harold becoming 'Warden' and Kate remaining Lady Supervisor and Matron, though she stops being mentioned in the directories and from this point disappears from publicity, standing in the shadow of her husband for the remainder of her life. The Retreat was licensed for 20 women and the regime they went through purported:

> to teach all how to be better housewives and also instruct them in various home industries, so that they may have an additional means of earning a livelihood... The whole treatment is carefully conducted upon a religious basis with a view to showing the inmates their sin and leading them by gentle means to higher things[23]

The Royal Victoria Home [RVH] was unusual. Most retreats were commercial operations, who admitted men who could afford to pay the fees. The RVH was for women, and unusually appears to have operated as a charity. Like other charities in Bristol it needed fundraising[24] to operate and claimed to be supported by such notables as

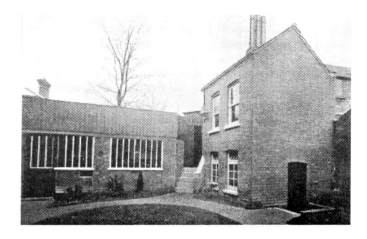

Figure 3.3: Laundry at Royal Victoria Home, Horfield

> the Duke and Duchess of Beaufort, the Duchess of Bedford, the Countess of Dudley, Lady Battersea and many others...the Home is the only Public Industrial or Charitable Institution built and established for this special work in the United Kingdom.[25]

The Royal Victoria Homes

Brentry became an Inebriate Institution because of a need to expand the Royal Victoria Home in Horfield.

> Although only of so recent establishment, the Home at Horfield has been twice enlarged, and the accommodation proving to be still insufficient, the Management determined to procure larger premises and to this end instructed its officers to search for a suitable property; with the result; at the end of November [1898], a property containing some 89 acres of land was procured, and the first week of January [1899] existing premises there-on were licensed for the reception of 50 retreat cases.[26]

The creation of the Brentry Extension of the RVH was more complicated than this brief description suggests. The decision to look for a site such as Brentry was determined by the 1898 Inebriates Act, [27] which created Inebriate Reformatories for the compulsory detention and treatment of inebriates. To work though, it needed a lot of new Inebriate Reformatories to be set up. The Act allowed councils to contribute to the maintenance of a retreat or a reformatory, but few were likely to be keen to incur the expense of setting them up. The charity of the RVH could not hope to have the money to set up a reformatory. The plan conceived was to set up a reformatory in which Councils bought what were effectively shares, so they were not frightened by having to put up large expenses.

In September 1898 the Rev. Burden sent out a flyer to councils asking them if they had considered their plans for the Inebriates Act and suggesting they might like to support plans to secure Brentry.[28] Gloucestershire County Council advised the promoters (the committee of the RVH) that the Council would only entertain proposals from a going concern, especially after they were told that 'the promoters' provided no money and gave no guarantee or undertaking of any kind.[29] Harold Burden also requested a lifetime appointment as warden and superintendent but this was flatly rejected.

The Rev. Burden first rented Brentry from the Millers in November 1898[30] and in the same month distributed a broad-sheet and brochure[31] advertising the particulars of Brentry in more detail and a proposal to set it up as the Brentry Extension of the RVH, as an Inebriate Reformatory. On the 9 January 1899[32] he licensed Brentry as an extension of the RVH. It was licensed as a retreat for 50 women and used only the old buildings so little work was needed.

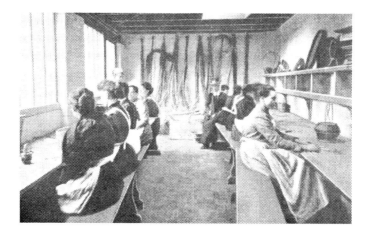

Figure 3.4: Basket weaving at the Royal Victoria Home, Horfield.

The main building was used for officers, staff and for 'the class of patients who can afford a higher fee' whilst the stable block was used for those 'whose friends can only afford to pay a smaller fee'.[33]

With this evidence that the site could be a 'going concern' and even though it was still empty, the Councils were approached for serious funding. In March 1899, Gloucestershire County Council convened a meeting of County Councils at the Guildhall London where it was agreed to proceed with the Brentry Plan[34] at a further meeting on the 12th April. Brentry was licensed as a Female Reformatory (for 75 women, operated jointly by Mr Burden and his wife Katherine) on the 31 March 1899[35] thus achieving the 'credit' of becoming the first reformatory ever licensed under the new Act.[36] At the April meeting a number of County Councils agreed to contribute a lump sum each to purchase the site and build residential blocks, in return for admitting rights and reduced payments for inmates.[37] The first woman inmate was admitted to Brentry on the 24 April 1899.[38]

By July seven councils had committed a total of £8000 to the project and on 26 July 1899 Mr Burden and Mr Edward Thomas formally purchased the Brentry Estate with its 82 acres. They paid the Millers £11,650 for Brentry, and £850 for a neighbouring 3 acres held by the Millers.[39] Rather oddly, they bought it using some council cash, but mainly using a £9000 mortgage supplied by the Millers,[40] which effectively meant that they were paying the Millers in instalments for the property.

On 28 July 1899, the scheme was legally set out by means of a trust deed.[41] When drafting this trust deed, the Burdens now asked for a 25 year appointment but they were refused as firmly as with the life appointment. The first Board Meeting under the Trust Deed was held at 45 Park Street, Bristol on Friday 4th August 1899. It carried the following resolutions:

> 5. That the Board places on record its recognition of the services gratuitously rendered by Mr E. Thomas in connection with the establishment of the Homes…
> 6. That the Board places on record its recognition of the services gratuitously rendered to the Homes by Dr Cotton of Horfield….
> 7. That the board desires to place on record its deep sense of the valuable and disinterested services performed by the Warden in connection with the establishment of the Homes and their management, under exceptionally difficult and trying circumstances. That the Board is of opinion that, with a view to the establishment of the Homes on a fair and permanent basis and to their success and extension, it is of the greatest importance that the permanent duties of the Warden should, as far as practicable, be secured.
> 8. That while the board has every intention to retain the valuable services of the Warden during his competency to fulfil the duties, it does not see its way to pledging the Board or the Warden to any fixed term of years. [Noted that he was appointed as warden by the Trust Deed].

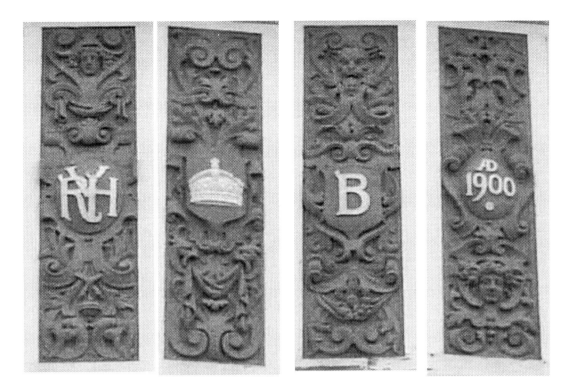

Figure 3.5: Plasterwork in the lower village at Brentry

> 9. That the question of an agreement with the Warden be referred to the General Purposes Committee for report at the next meeting, with special reference to the question of pension and notice.[42]

The tone of this resolution suggests that the board was reluctant to appoint the Rev Burden for life as he was not in the best of health. He was certainly ill the following year, when the post of Assistant Superintendent was upgraded to Deputy Warden.[43]

The institution was called the "Royal Victoria Homes, Brentry, Near Bristol", with the approval of Queen Victoria. The name was emblazoned into the plaster of the new buildings (Figure 3.3). The trust deed created the Institution as a joint venture between the Management of the Horfield Royal Victoria Home (known as the Promoters) and the founding councils, with the property being transferred from Mr Thomas and the Rev. Burden to 12 Trustees. The councils provided 6 trustees, as did the promoters. The six Horfield trustees included such notables as Lewis and Francis James Fry, the Bishop of Bristol and Sir Michael Hicks Beach, the Chancellor of the Exchequer. Each group contributed 12 members of the Board of Management, and the first chairman of this Board was to be Captain Belfield, the Chairman of the Horfield RVH. The deed sets out that future subscribing councils would also contribute a member to this Board, with the intention of eventually taking over the running of the reformatory. This is indeed what occurred, as by 1901 23 councils had subscribed, so that the council members outnumbered the Horfield members by 2 to 1. As the Inspector reported:

> Each of the … Councils has appointed a representative on the Board of Management, which is now composed chiefly of such members. The whole undertaking has, therefore, virtually become an institution controlled by public bodies.[44]

In the summer of 1899 both the RVH and Brentry required conversion to expand as reformatories and this necessitated a temporary cessation of admissions. During December 1899 Brentry only held one female inebriate[45] though 46 had been admitted to the Retreat side during the year.[46]

The building work at Brentry was to prove extensive. Mr Burden started with quick conversions. The Stables were converted for 75 women. Then the two cottages in the lower village were converted to a block (block M in Figure 4.1) along with creating some workshops and a wash-house, to be able to licence the lower village for 30 males on 13 December 1899. The first male inmate was admitted on 6 February 1900.[47] After this there were some purpose built cottages: two cottages were built for the lower village [blocks N & O] and the design reused in the upper village [blocks A & B].

> Three separate certificates have been granted to this Board, one for the female, and one for the male portions of Brentry, and a third for Horfield. The latter house, being considered unsuitable for full certification, permission has been granted for its use as a reception house [for women] for the main institution. The three divisions are being conducted jointly, as the RVH's.[48]

The main building programme now started in earnest, financed by the new subscriptions from Councils. The main features of the colony were completed by the end of 1900. It was then licensed as a Reformatory for 150 Females and 111 Males. It was also licensed as a Retreat for 25 of each sex,[49] but it was decided not to admit Retreat cases 'until more distinct and isolated buildings exist for the reception of such cases'.[50] These never seem to have occurred, and no more Retreat cases seem to have been admitted. Brentry now operated as a Licensed Reformatory called The Royal Victoria Homes, Brentry.

Notes

[1] The best accounts are in Roy M. MacLeod: 'The Edge of Hope: Social Policy and Chronic Alcoholism 1870 - 1900.' *J.Hist.Medicine* 1967 (22): 215-245, and L. Radzinowicz & R Hood: *A History of English Criminal Law and its Administration from 1750. Volume 5.* London: Stevens & Sons, 1986. Chapter 9.

[2] Mary Carpenter *Our Convicts* (1863) vol 2, p314-23 (quoted in Radzinowicz p301)

[3] P McCandless: 'Curses of Civilization': Insanity and Drunkenness in Victorian Britain. *British Journal of Addiction* 1984. **79:**49-58.

[4] T Laycock: *The Social and Political Relations of Drunkenness.* Edinburgh,1857

[5] quoted in Radinowicz *op cit* page 294-5.

[6] Trevor May *An Economic and Social History of Britain 1760- 1970.* Essex, Harlow: Longmans, 1987 page 134.

[7] MacLeod *op. cit.* Cites that the incidence of arrests rose by 50% between 1867 and 1876. (p215, n15).

[8] *An Act to facilitate the control and care of Habitual Drunkards.* 42 & 43 Vict. c.19 (1879)

[9] *The Times* 17 June 1878 - quoted by MacLeod

[10] *An Act to amend the Habitual Drunkards' Act, 1879.*

[11] Radzinowicz (*op cit*) p301

[12] *An Act to provide for the Treatment of Habitual Inebriates.* 1898 and *An Act to Amend the Inebriates' Act, 1898.* 1899

[13] see Carpenter P.K.: Rev. Harold Nelson Burden & Katherine Mary Burden - pioneers of Inebriate Reformatories and Mental Deficiency Institutions. *Journal of the Royal Society of Medicine* 1996 **89:**205-9.

[14] Obituary, Clevedon Mercury 8 November 1919, reprinted in J Jancar *Research at Stoke Park - Mental Handicap (1930 - 1980)* Bristol, Frenchay Health Authority 1981

[15] Carpenter P. K.: Missionaries with the Hopeless? Inebriety, mental deficiency and the Burdens. *British Journal of Learning Disabilities* 2000 **28:**60-4.

[16] Wright & Co Bristol Directory for 1896 & 1897 which show his address as Woodside, 132 Chesterfield Road, Bristol.

[17] Letter by Edward Thomas to *Bristol Mercury* circa Sept 1902. Copy at *B.R.O.:* 40359/B/8

[18] Fourteenth annual report of the Inspector of Retreats, 1893: BPP: 1894 [C.7519]XXI.695 page 8.

[19] Letter by Edward Thomas to *Bristol Mercury* circa Sept 1902, copy at Bristol Record Office, Uncatalogued deposition for Brentry.

[20] Katherine's Obituary - *op cit*

[21] J Wright & Co's Bristol and Clifton Directory, 1897 Bristol: J Wright, 1897 pg697-8.

[22] Printed minutes of Brentry Board of Management 28 Sept 1903, page 10

[23] Entry for RVH, Wrights & Co Bristol Directory 1898

[24] For a description of one such event see Penelope's Diary in *Bath and County Graphic* 7 June 1897 - quoted in G Davis, P Bonsall: *Bath a New History.* Keele Univ Press 1996 page 85.

[25] On header of the RVH, *GRO:* CJ1/C1

[26] 19th report of the Inspector of Retreats for Habitual Drunkards. 1898. BPP:1899 [C.9451] xii 731 pg217

[27] An Act to provide for the Treatment of Habitual Inebriates 1898

[28] *GLRO:* CJ1/C1

[29] CJ1/C1 undated memorandum but probably relates to this period.

[30] Annual accounts for Brentry quote cost of renting prior to date of purchase and the interest prior to opening came to £259; for Start of November - see 19th Annual report of the Inspector of Retreats ... for 1898; 1899 xii 731 [C.9451] entry for the RVH.

[31] BRO 40359 and Bristol Reference Library accession numbers 31219-22

[32] Twentieth report of the Inspectors of Retreats ... under the Inebriates Act, 1899. BPP: 1901 [Cd.445] x 735 - copy of application have from GLRO:CJ1/C1

[33] *19th report of the Inspector of Retreats for Habitual Drunkards. 1898.* BPP: 1899 [C.9451] xii 731

[34] 40359 - copy in tin box

[35] *GLRO*:CJ1/C1 has application amended from that of RVH.

[36] *Twentieth report of the Inspectors of Retreats and the first report of the Inspector of Certified Reformatories under the Inebriates Act, 1899:* 1901 [Cd.445] x 735. Page 31-2

[37] *BRO* 40359, and Bristol Reference Library Accn No 31218

[38] Annual report of Board of Management for 1899, page 10

[39] deeds of conveyance both dated 26 July 1898, held by Bevan Ashford Solrs.

[40] Mortgage to Audley Montague Miller, dated 27 July 1898 at Bevan Ashfords; In the first annual report of Brentry, Captain Belfield the Chairman reported that the site was purchased for £13000, and that there is a £10,000 mortgage on the property.(*Proceedings of the Board of Management ... June 25th 1900 and Annual Report...* Page 7)

[41] Trust deed dated 28 July 1899, copies at *BRO* 40359, original held by Bevan Ashfords Solrs

[42] BRO: 40359/B/8(a) Printed Proceedings

[43] BRO: 40359/B/8(a) Printed report of committee 8 Feb 1902.

[44] *Twentieth report of the Inspectors of Retreats and the first report of the Inspector of Certified Reformatories under the Inebriates Act, 1899:* 1901 [Cd.445] x 735

[45] *Twentieth report of the Inspectors of Retreats ... under the Inebriates Act, 1899:* 1901 [Cd.445] x 735

[46] Wardens report for 1899, *Proceedings ... Board of Management ... March 26th 1900 ...,* page 8; Eighteen women were admitted to the retreat side during 1899 according to the *Twentieth report of the Inspectors of Retreats ... under the Inebriates Act, 1899.* (BPP: 1901 [Cd.445] x 735) The 46 may therefore include the admissions to both Horfield and Brentry sites.

[47] Annual Report of Board of Management for 1899, page 10

[48] *Twentieth report of the Inspectors of Retreats and the first report of the Inspector of Certified Reformatories under the Inebriates Act, 1899:* 1901 [Cd.445] x 735. Page 31-2

[49] *Annual report of Inspector 1900*: 1902 [Cd. 811] xii 599

[50] Annual Report of Board of Management for 1899 *op cit* page 8

The Royal Victoria Homes (Brentry)

The Brentry Reformatory was now the largest in the country and was described in glowing detail in the Inebriate Reformatory Inspector's annual report for 1900.[1] (Figure 4.1)

> When last under notice it was described as consisting of two distinct sections, Horfield and Brentry. The former only received a modified certificate, enabling the buildings concerned to be used as a reception house for the main institution, not as a reformatory for the permanent residence of inmates. This portion may now be dismissed from further consideration with the information that it remains unaltered and is serving the purpose indicated.
>
> Brentry on the other hand, is greatly enlarged and improved in efficiency. When first certified as a reformatory the Brentry division consisted of a large mansion and outbuilding, the whole of which had been so altered and rebuilt as to be capable of accommodating 75 female inmates [marked 'J'-in Figure 4.1 – the old stables, cost of work £2600 – see also Figures 4.3 & 4.4]. In addition there was a block of cottages, distinct and distant from the main building, similarly modified and adapted for the reception of 30 male inmates ['M' -cost £645, Figure 4.5]. These together constituted the male and female sides for the institution.
>
> Recent additions to the female side have doubled the available accommodation, and have added largely to facilities for good management. These mainly consist of: (1) four semi-detached cottages ['A','B','N','O'- total cost £6300 – Figures 4.6 & 4.7],[2] (2) a new entrance block containing offices and rooms in which visitors can interview inmates ['H' – Figure 4.8]; (3) a well-designed infirmary [for women only!] capable of accommodating 16 patients with every necessary convenience for the treatment of the sick ['C']; (4) a recreation hall with space for seating 200 people and fitted with a stage and dressing rooms ['D' – Figure 4.9]; (5) an engine house and electric generating station ['G' – Figure 4.10]; (6) a well arranged laundry with all modern appliances ['I' – Figure 4.11] and (7) improved accommodation for the control of refractory cases. ... in addition... enlarged kitchen [Figure 4.12], increased dining accommodation, better officers quarters,... whole inst fitted with electric light, and a complete telephone system... The grounds surrounding the houses have been artistically laid out...
>
> Male side ... has also been object of additions but owing to the smaller demand for accommodation, to a less degree... two blocks of buildings similar in all respects to those provided for the accommodation of females. A reception house, some isolation rooms for refractory cases ['K' the basement a police station, with cells for refractory cases, the top two floors for reception - cost £1010 – Figure 4.13] and a block of workshops ['L'] complete the list of more important changes. ...   [two more pages of encouragement][3]

In addition a corrugated Iron Workshop['E'] had been built on the site of the 1930's Concert Hall, and the boundary walls built cost £811.[4]

In addition the old kitchen courtyard, forming the space between the stables and main building, was roofed in 1900 to create a hall[5] [Figure 4.14]. The main house was used exclusively for the officers, with the upstairs part of the main house being mainly used for the Burdens, though they continued to use the Horfield RVH as their official address.[6] The expansion in staff also required the purchase of 9 cottages close by to the site for their accommodation.[7]

The Rev. Burden and his wife were paid £300 per annum jointly. The Managers first tried to employ Dr Cotton, the medical officer for the Horfield RVH, as the Medical Officer for Brentry offering him the same terms as a medical officer in the Prison Service. He declined, and Dr Ormerod, the medical officer for the neighbouring Barton Regis Workhouse [now Southmead Hospital] was appointed by December 1899[8] at £150 per annum. He had taken over the practice of his father, Dr H. Ormerod, who had been on the staff of the B.R.I.[9] before moving to Westbury and taking on the Barton Regis Workhouse. With the expansion of the licence in 1900, a deputy Warden, Lt-Col. W. G. Small, 'late of the H.M. 59th Regiment'[10] was appointed, along with an expanded male staff. The Post of Deputy Warden was originally

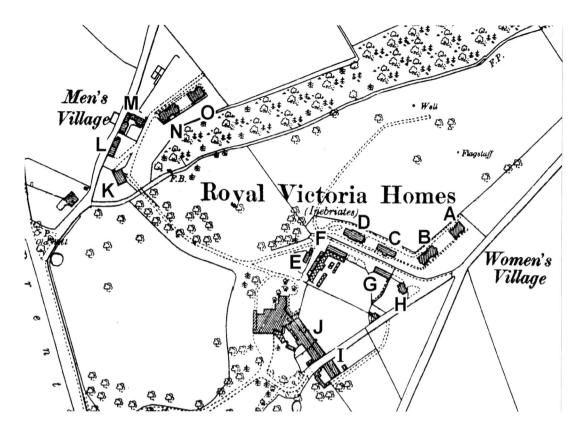

Figure 4.1: The Brentry Site 1903 – wards are lettered according to 1900 description.

planned to be that of Assistant Superintendent, but this was upgraded due to Mr Burden being ill.

The new reformatory published a pamphlet[11] and a brochure of photographs[12] (from which this chapter is illustrated) to advertise its existence and purpose. The brochure includes a photograph of the chief staff of the Institution (Figure 4.2) which at its centre has a moustached Rev. Harold Burden and his wife. This is the only image known of the pair of them together. The other officers shown must include Dr Ormerod(wearing a boater?) and Lt-Colonel Small (a bowler hat?) but which they are in the photograph is more conjectural. The pamphlet emphasised the skills of its chief officers:

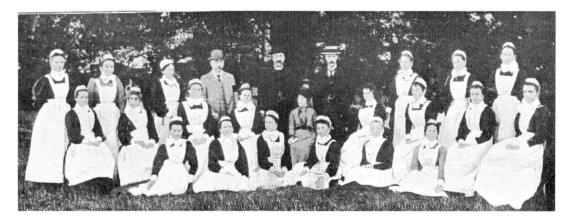

Figure 4.2: The Chief Officers and some of the female staff of the Institution 1901. Rev. Burden is in the middle with his wife in front of him.

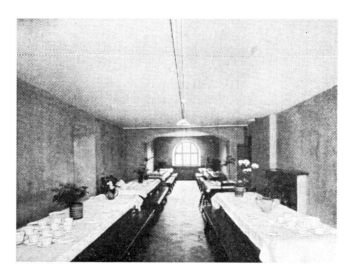

Figure 4.3: Women's dining room in the Stable Block

> The Warden [Rev H N Burden] has been engaged for years in similar work and has made this his life's study. The deputy warden [Colonel Small] has served Her late Majesty with distinction in every rank on officer can hold, from a Subaltern up to Lieut-Colonel; The Medical Officer [Dr H L Ormerod, MD] has had many years' experience as Resident Surgeon in a large Infirmary, as well as private practice. The Lady Superintendent [Mrs K. M. Burden] has spent almost a life-time in work amongst the class of persons mostly sent to the Homes, while one Assistant Matron has had eight years' Infirmary experience, and the other several years at a large Workhouse. ... [In addition there are]: a Chaplain ... Senior Male Officer, Store and Book Keepers, Officers in charge of Kitchens, Laundry, Baths, Workrooms, Out-door Working Parties and other departments, Assistant Day and Night Officers, trained Nurses, Attendants and others. An Engineer-Foreman, Farm Bailiff, Head Gardener, Police Sergeant, Police Constables, and other Officers.[13]

The reformatory generally received adulatory reports in the press[14] and in the annual reports of the Inebriate Reformatory Inspector Dr Branthwaite, who later became a close friend of the Burdens. Though Dr Branthwaite comments on the lack of occupation in his report for 1901 his criticisms are followed by congratulations:

> I refer to the necessity for the more constant occupation of inmates. Brentry is not alone amongst reformatories in falling short in this direction, but it is more evident at Brentry than elsewhere because of the greater number of persons under detention. ... I am aware that much is done already, and that regular institution work - the manufacture of clothing, laundry work, gardening, &c. - take up the time of many inmates; but there are sundry others who are only partly employed, and who should be fully occupied.
> ...Brentry is an excellent institution... It has an excellent Board of managers, who take an active personal interest in the success of the institution, and a Superintendent, whose equal in energy, ability, and forethought it would be extremely difficult to find.[15]

The *Rules for the Domestic Management and Discipline of the Certified Inebriate Reformatories at Brentry and Horfield*[16] shows a tough life - every inmate was to be searched on admission and whenever needed. The food was to be 'plain and wholesome' and the inmates' day lasted from 6.45am to 9.30pm, with physical drill, prayers and 7 hours of work each day. Inmates might be allowed to wear their own clothes but had to keep their rooms, utensils cloths and bedding clean, neat and well cared for. All inmates had to work outdoors for part of the day when the weather

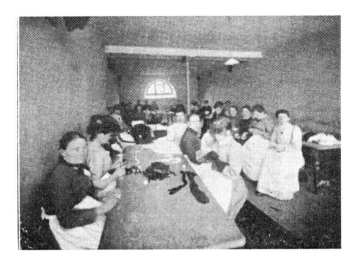

Figure 4.4: Women mending, in workshop in the Stable Block

was fine. In their leisure time they had to keep themselves actively employed and 'in no case are they to sit idly about'. All visits, even from officials, could only occur with the written permission of the Warden or the Inspector and must always occur in the sight of an Officer of the Homes. Every letter to and from the inmates had to be read by the Warden, except for letters to the Secretary of State or Inspector. Disciplinary offences included such acts as to 'make any objectionable noise, give any unnecessary trouble or make repeated groundless complaints' and could lead to the Warden ordering the loss of diet, of liberty or of any other privilege. There was a bread and gruel diet for the troublemakers.

The dietary of Brentry was simple and in modern terms was extremely unappetising. It was however, probably better than what the inmates were used to. In 1910 the provisions for Brentry cost an average of 3s 8d per inmate per week, excluding the food produced on site. In 1911 it was claimed that in the community single working women would spend between 3s and 6s on food each week, and that working families would average 3s to 4s per person per week.[17]

The First Financial Crisis

The adulatory reports of Dr Branthwaite omitted to mention that by the end of 1900 Brentry was already in a financial crisis. Though the councils had reserved 194 beds, only 58 were occupied and the revenue gap was untenable.[18]

The vacancies on the female side were soon filled, and the female side was further expanded by a 'temporary building' during June 1901[19] on the site later occupied by 'C' Block or Wellington Villa. This building was later named 'Warwick' (Figure 5.8). By December 1901 there were 156 female inmates[20] with 37 female officers[21] and the female side was returning a profit.

The millstone was the Male side. Though there was 111 places licensed for men and 15 staff, there was only an average of 16 men resident in early 1901, and this figure reached only 32 by the end of 1901 despite much hard work. The financial difficulties were relayed to the Inebriates Acts Department at the Home Office, presumably with a request for increased State subsidy, but this drew a damning confidential letter from Branthwaite, sent out to the managers:

> The points that appeal to me are (1) the character, (2) the number, and (3) the expense of your staff. You must surely have realized, long since, that more difficulty was going to be experienced in obtaining Male committals than Female. ... This being so, why did you make such extensive additions to your staff? It appears that on October 1st last you had ten officers with an aggregate expenditure on salaries of £585 per annum. During the next three months these figures increased so that on January 1st 1901, you show fifteen male officers

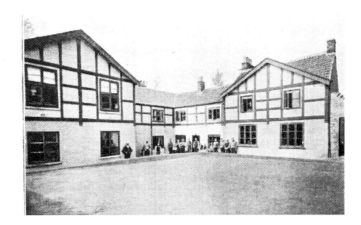

Figure: 4.5: The first Men's cottage

whose stipends collectively amount to £1150 per annum ... Fifteen male officers to control about 20 men appears to me ridiculous. You appear further to have appointed a highly-paid officer to superintend a still quite small Institution, when in my opinion such an appointment was quite unwarranted.

When the Reformatory was first started some excellent regulations, (including model arrangements for a male staff) were approved by the Secretary of State, but do not seem to have been given even a trial.... In short, I consider that your male staff is unnecessarily good, it is too large and overpaid.[22]

Branthwaite recommended a change in the male staff with only 7 staff for up to 50 residents as quite adequate. However the male inmates had been proving rather troublesome. Some of the earlier resolutions included advice to the courts that 'violent and malicious persons should not be committed to Brentry'[23] and Col. Small, responding to Branthwaite's comments, stated that

the present establishment is the minimum necessary to ensure efficiency, the maintenance of order ... the majority of the Male inmates are men who are only kept in their present state of control and discipline by the knowledge that there is always available sufficient physical force to restrain them. The documentary history of these men shows them to have been the most troublesome characters of the localities from which they have been sent....That as the cells have been almost continuously occupied by inmates who have been most insubordinate and violent, it has been conclusively shown that the numbers of the Police have been no more than equal to the demand made upon them by the custody of these men,...[24]

This was borne out by a letter written by him on 20 June 1901 saying that 6 male inmates had been steadily fomenting discontent and on the 7th June had indulged in an 'almost mutinous refusal to work, unless they received special remuneration for it.' Mr Burden appealed to the Secretary of State and the Home Office opened a portion of Cardiff Prison as a State Inebriate reformatory for the transfer of the ring-leaders.[25] Then in January 1903 two men absconded but were recaptured.[26] Another inmate absconded two weeks later, climbing through a window at night and making the warden order the barring of the windows.[27] However the females were no angels. In October 1902 the warden reported that 'very offensive' letters had been found, written by the females to the male inmates.[28]

It is fair to say that the financial solution of Branthwaite would have not cured the overspend. The accounts of 1901 show a £3,300 deficit on a £8,600 turnover. The total staff salary was only £2700 (the male officers cost £982 and females £665). Sacking all the staff would not have covered the deficit.

The Reformatory was suffering from a general social problem of the inebriate acts. Unlike with the Retreats, the Reformatories were being filled with paupers who had been convicted. The men generally had pauper dependants. Magistrates choosing between fining a man or sending him

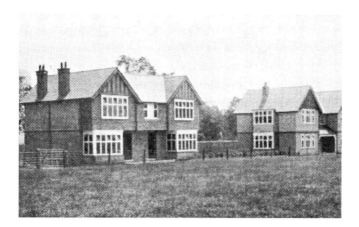

Figure 4.6: The Women's Cottages

to a reformatory for three years, or to prison for seven days would have been very aware of the effect on the rest of the family and the likelihood that they would end up paupers on the poor rates. So though there were four times more men than women being convicted of drinking offences, many more women than men were being sent to the inebriate reformatories. The men who the magistrates did commit to the longer sentence of the reformatory were likely to have already separated from their families due to their behaviour, or to be hardened, recurrent offenders. Women seem to have been sent away more easily, possibly because they were seen as failing their role as a mother – a 'considerable number of women [sent to reformatories were] convicted of neglecting their children'.[29] In addition women were less likely to be able to pay the fines.[30] The people attending the Retreats were still rarely poor and mainly men.

The financial losses at Brentry could not be borne for long. By August 1901 the Board was overdrawn at the bank. Letters of appeal had been sent to the Secretary of State but his reply simply asked what steps had been taken to implement Branthwaite's recommendations? At this time though, the State was already paying over twice what the councils were for the inmates in Brentry. The Board agreed to dismiss Col Small and such other officers as the Managers considered could be immediately dispensed with and the contributing councils were asked to pay 6d per reserved bed, whether occupied or not.[31] A special meeting on the 23 September 1901 resolved to take out a further mortgage of £3000 on the Property, but this proved impossible. The Board resolved to explore closing the male side but found only the Church Army and Association for the Care of Inebriate Persons were interested and their terms were unacceptable.[32]

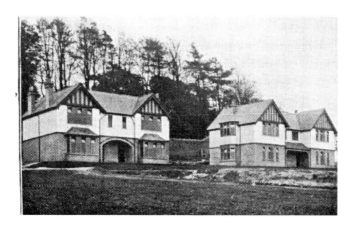

Figure 4.7: The Men's Cottages

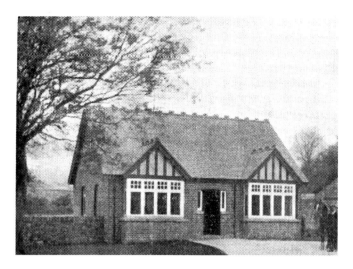

Figure 4.8: The Enquiry Office.

On the 9th December, it was decided to see if the Contributing Councils would bail out Brentry at the price of fully taking it over.[33] A committee was set up to explore this and to solve the financial crisis: It revised the management structure and prevented Col. Small from challenging his dismissal by saying he had never been properly appointed.

At the next Annual General meeting of 24 March 1902, Sir Henry Mather Jackson, the representative of Monmouthshire, took over the Chairmanship of Brentry from Captain Belfield, (the nominee of the Horfield RVH) and Capt. Belfield resigned from the Board of Management at the next meeting. Though rescue seemed likely, financial pressures continued, with unexpectedly large bills from the architect, from the builder sinking the well (which was twice the anticipated depth); repeated calls by the Roman Catholic Chaplain for a salary; and high rate demands from the local parishes. In addition a fire in the main building on the 4 October 1902 destroyed 3 officers bedrooms and a portion of the roof[34] of the three storey extension. Repairs were covered by the fire insurance, but the committee accepted the need to in addition rebuild the whole area. They altered the kitchen on the Ground Floor and the floors above it, adding a third storey to improve the staff accommodation and make quarters for the Second Officer.[35]. They replaced the burnt wooden staircase with a stone one (which remains as the staircase for the three storey part of the building) but added a wooden one above the kitchen to access the new third floor. At the same time they authorised as a necessity, the building of a new kitchen. This was built during 1904[36] and remained in use for the rest of the century.

The contributing councils were asked to all contribute an extra £250 for every £1000 initially contributed. They protested, but agreed.[37] The price was a new Charity Scheme approved in November 1903 by the Charity Commissioners. This authorised the increased contributions, changed the name of the Colony from the *Royal Victoria Homes - Brentry extension*, to the *Brentry Certified Inebriate Reformatory*[38] and granted the councils perpetual rights, rather than the 25 years originally agreed. The councils paid up £6000 and a capital sum of £5171 was transferred to the Maintenance account to bring it out of debt.[39] At the same time, on 10 November 1903, the licence was reduced to 105 women and 135 men.[40] The total number was reduced because the Government decided both to pay less to reformatories larger than 200 and that Brentry was one reformatory and not two as the councils hoped. [41]. Though it had been the male side that was the financial millstone, the managers realised that there were virtually no other reformatories for men in the country, and saw this side as having a future.

The crisis was almost over. With the reduced staffing the receipts exceeded expenditure during the first half of 1903.[42] Though the male side had still only reached 52 inmates at the end of 1903, the place was full by the end of the March 1904 quarter. The links with the Horfield RVH

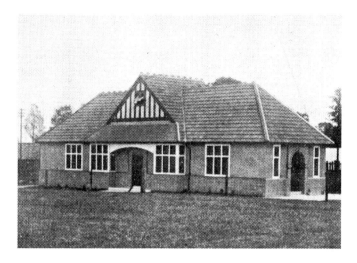

Figure 4.9: the Women's recreation hall.

were by now almost totally severed: the Chairman, Treasurer and Solicitor appointed by them had been replaced and their other board members had resigned or died and not been replaced.

The closure of Horfield RVH

The Brentry extension of the RVH emasculated its parent house. Whilst Brentry's income came from the commercial revenue for its reformatory beds, the Horfield RVH was a charity originally set up to provide a retreat and a home for poor convict women. With the creation of Brentry as a reformatory the RVH had bizarrely become the reception house for the women entering Brentry. It was now part of a more commercial venture and inevitably the philanthropists stopped donating money to it. It was in financial difficulties within a year.[43] On the 26 March 1900 the Brentry Board (with its Horfield nominees) resolved to consider taking it over. However nothing happened. The Horfield committee decided to force the issue, realising that they had no formal contract with Brentry. In December 1900 the Rev Burden informed the Brentry House Committee that Horfield House would close on at the end of the month and Brentry would be without a receiving house for females. He also said that they were not able to proceed in building a receiving house at Brentry for several months. Mrs Davies and Mr Fedden (who were Horfield RVH nominees) proposed that the Brentry Board took over the Horfield House for 6 months or more.[44] Then it was proposed to the Brentry Board that they accepted an agreement to take over the Horfield Premises on a quarterly basis, at a rent of £40 per annum, plus rates and taxes.[45] The agreement was signed and Horfield continued as the receiving house for women. However Capt. Belfield later wrote:

> I do not think you would find on the minutes any reference made to the £40 bargain between Brentry and Horfield. The same was common knowledge, often talked over, and personally I was against it as I did not consider it would benefit Brentry.[46]
> During the time that I was Chairman I was always "at" Mr Burden to put down everything on the minutes, and so have something definite to refer to. I well remember Mr B. bringing before us the matter of renting the Horfield Home for £40 annually and though I personally objected to it, thinking it was not required, it was carried; this surely should be on the minutes, and Mr Burden ought to be able to give you every possible information.[47]

There continued to be problems with the payments, as Brentry's financial problems escalated. The matter came to a head after a further year when the committee set up to solve Brentry's financial crisis reported in January 1902:

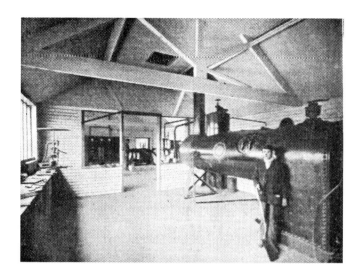

Figure 4.10: The Power Station

22: We cannot conclude this portion of our report without a reference to the case of the Home at Horfield, the existence of which came upon most of us as a surprise and upon all of us as most unsatisfactory.

It appears that there exists at Horfield, a small Home with 25 beds, which was the origin of the present Homes, but is quite distinct from them and not under the management of the Board. Without any sanction from this Board and without their knowledge as a Board, this home has been used as a Receiving House for the Female Inebriates who are kept there for some three weeks before being admitted to the Homes at Brentry. The staff are Officers of Brentry Homes, and the expenses are paid by the Brentry Homes, though the Warden only allows the cost of the Inmates there to amount to the average costs of those in Brentry Homes themselves, bearing any extra cost himself. It further appears that last year "to meet the wishes of the Horfield Board" an agreement was entered into by the Managers, by which the Horfield Home was taken at a rent of £40 a year and rates and taxes. No report of this transaction was ever made to the Brentry Board; probably, the Warden thinks owing to an oversight of his own, and though no rent has in fact been paid the agreement should not be recognised but should be cancelled and fresh arrangements be made for a Receiving House at Brentry.

Edward Thomas, on behalf of the Horfield Home tried for some time to obtain some rental from Brentry but to no avail. Canon Parker, the chairman of the Brentry finance committee, insisted that the agreement signed in January 1901 was wholly unauthorised.[48] He does not give a reason for saying this and one must assume his claim was based on financial necessity, but the minutes show that the committee had authorised the drawing up of an agreement for consideration, but had not authorised that the agreement be signed.

In July 1902 the Horfield Committee decided to sell the house, as all applications for the rent had been ignored by the Brentry management committee.[49] The Horfield RVH Board of Management formerly asked for money from the Rev. Burden, saying they had 'discovered' he was using the RVH as an extension of Brentry with patients being admitted there from Brentry. They also gave him notice to vacate his residence in the RVH.[50] The Management also asked for money from Brentry for the accommodation of the people who had been placed at Horfield. The Rev. Canon Parker replied that Brentry would pay by the head at Brentry costs and if this was too little Mr Burden was sort out the difference [as it was he who had signed the contract].[51] Canon Parker noted later (in August) that the Rev Burden had 'unbeknown to us' recently opened Horfield and there were again several inmates in it.[52] One assumes this happened as there was

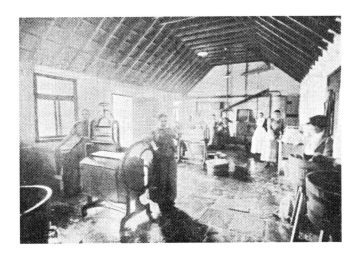

Figure 4.11: The Washing Room

still no reception house at Brentry for women, and the staff had no option but to use Horfield, but it was convenient for the Brentry Board to officially be unaware of the use.

The Horfield RVH Building was advertised for sale on the 24 September 1902[53] and was bought by the Burdens. In November the Rev Burden wrote that his purchase of the Horfield Home contained the condition 'the vendors abandon all claim for rent of the property' so ending the dispute over the rent.[54]

Mr Burden had a loyalty to the old Horfield RVH and kept it open as a reformatory and then as a 'holiday home' for 'mental defective women' until after his death. It was sold by his Trustees in 1933 and is now a block of flats.

The fall out from the loss of the Horfield RVH was the resignation of the Burdens. The Rev Burden had taken much of the blame for the financial crisis, along with the original board of management, but had been particularly blamed for the dispute with the Horfield RVH. In March 1902, after the loss of Lt-Col. Small, Mr Burden wrote to the Board of Management requesting the appointment of some more senior staff. He said that both he and his wife worked an average of 13 hours every day, excluding night calls, and they had been absent from the Site for a total of only 18 nights over 3 years [though he was still giving the Horfield Home as his address].[55] He wrote again in February 1903, and at a special meeting held on the 19 February 1903 announced his intention to resign as Warden. This he did on the 30 June but was appointed Honorary Secretary at the Annual General Meeting of 23 March 1903, when great thanks were expressed to him and his wife.[56] Soon afterwards, in February 1904, the mortgage to the Millers was cleared by the Board of Management who took over the mortgage liability from Messrs Thomas and Burden.[57]

Though Mr Burden stopped being the Warden, he still was very influential. He remained its Secretary. The Burdens reused the RVH as a reformatory and rented a series of other properties around England to create the *National Institutions for Inebriates.* By 1904 the *National Institutions* controlled over 450 beds. Their central offices included Brentry in their annual registers, which still survive.[58] These reveal much movement between Brentry and the *National Institutions'* reformatories. In total, the *National Institutions* paid for more of the inebriates at Brentry than did all the Contributing Councils.[59] The use of Brentry by the *National Institutions* probably kept it viable, as it enabled the use of vacant reserved beds, knowing the *Institutions* could remove its people to other reformatories when a council wanted to use its reserved bed.

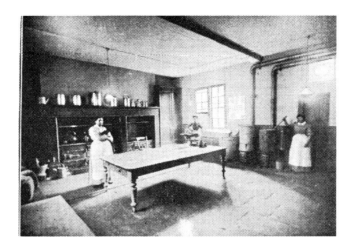

Figure 4.12: the Kitchen. (the old kitchen in the main house)

The Burdens later developed Mental Defective Colonies at Stoke Park and Whittington Hall and when the Rev. Burden died in 1930 his personal estate was £150,000 and the renamed *National Institutions for Persons Requiring Care and Control [NIPRCC]* owned property worth at least a further £400,000. Brentry seems to have been his first experience of having a major dispute with his management committee. It also reveals that committees became frustrated with his tendency not to record what was agreed. He continued to have great difficulty working with committees and later on was said to find them a nuisance.

The continuing work with Inebriates

The loss of the Horfield RVH as a receiving house meant that a new receiving house for women was needed for Brentry. It was built in 1903[60] and the new Kitchens completed the following year. The post of Warden was replaced by that of Superintendent - 'the title given to the Chief Officer in all similar Institutions'.[61] Dr David Fleck of Caterham Asylum was appointed and took up his post on the 30 June 1903 as joint Superintendent and medical officer. A few junior staff resigned after his arrival. Dr Ormerod stopped being medical officer, but was appointed 'Consulting Medical Officer', so that he could cover in Dr Fleck's absence.[62] Of the two assistant matrons: Miss Cottle was premoted to matron at £75 p.a. and Miss Hopkins had her salary increased to £60 p.a.. There were also further changes at Board level. In April 1904 Mather Jackson resigned as Chairman as he found attending the House Committees too onerous. Canon Parker replaced him,[63] but died in 1908, when Mather Jackson returned as Chairman and held the post for almost another 30 years.[64]

Brentry continued to be one of the few male reformatories and this side continued to expand, though there was no more building in the lower village. By the end of 1905, the lower village had overflowed, and some of the 100 men in residence had to be housed in the old female rooms in the stables, close to the female village. During 1906 a new block was built in the men's village to provide dormitories, a hall, workshops and additional bathing facilities. This was built by the inmates at a cost of £1200 (Figure 5.2 – block marked 'A', now named 'Lewis House') and has '1906' inscribed on the eaves, though it was completed in 1907. In addition the well was yet further deepened to try and obtain sufficient water for the expanding population.

On the 17 June 1906 there was a second mutiny at Brentry:

> an inmate named William Phillips in the male receiving house,... attacked the Assistant Superintendent and struck him a severe blow in the eye, 5 others joined in the disturbance and assaulted the officers, the 6 men then commenced breaking the furniture and windows, their conduct became so violent that Police were sent for from Henbury and Westbury-on-Trym.....[the four policemen who

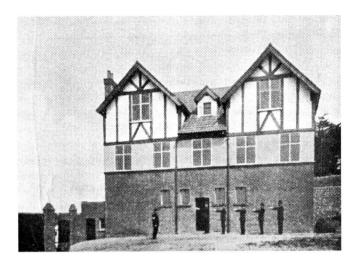

Figure 4.13: The Men's Reception Block with Police Station underneath (and police)

> attended] remained until order was restored, the 6 men were then in the Cells. At the time of the outbreak there were 22 men in the receiving house but only the 6 appears to take part in the disturbance. ... [the next morning] the 6 men were still in the Cells. I examined the receiving ward and found 5 chairs and 126 panes of glass broken. The Supt informed me that he had communicated with the Home Secretary and was awaiting his instructions.[65]

The men were all prosecuted and removed and two special constables were appointed for a time, paid for by the managers of Brentry,[66] to reduce the anxieties of the neighbourhood. The Board wrote to the Home Secretary, bewailing the reduction in the Treasury grant that made looking after these inmates even more difficult. One of the board members has written in the margins:

> The whole question is can these Reformatories be carried on at the cost suggested by the Home Secy - if not, they will have to be closed & the Act will prove a failure.[67]

The Treasury did not restore its subsidy and though Brentry was full, it was again running in debt in July 1907. Further financial troubles came with an outbreak of Typhoid, with 28 cases and two deaths between September 1906 and November 1907. Eleven cases were staff or their families. There were exhaustive and expensive checks of the drains, well, and dairy herd. The dairy and sewerage system were improved but to no avail. Eventually a visitor went down with typhoid after a brief visit to Brentry where he had only tea and sandwiches.[68] From this mishap was traced the carrier who worked in the diary - 'Inmate X', the 'Typhoid Mary' of Brentry. The managers were unsure how to deal with this infectious lady and asked the Secretary of State to allow her discharge or remove her to prison, but he declined.[69]

David Fleck started to organise Brentry along similar lines to a lunatic asylum. He brought in three 'classes' of inmate on each side, with an admission, upper and lower class, each with differing 'accommodation, food, work, and rewards, positions of trust, liberties allowed and other minor privileges.'[70] The mark system for work was revised, allowing inmates to earn up to 7d per week depending on their work. On the male side, the Refomatory made and sold wooden garden furniture and utensils and a catalogue of their work survives.[71]

In one annual report Dr Fleck describes the discharge and aftercare arrangements for Inmates:

> For each monthly meeting of the House Committee a report is prepared, showing the names of all cases due for discharge during the succeeding month, with the person or association responsible for their aftercare, and for sending reports to the Reformatory. Each case discharged is provided with a change of

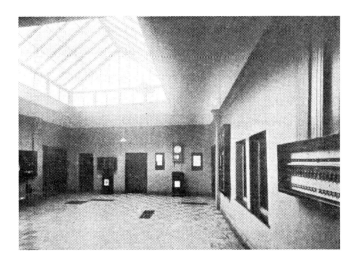

Figure 4.14: The Central Hall, formed by roofing in the back courtyard

decent clothing, given 5/-, and placed on the train at Bristol, provided they do not belong to that City, with their fare paid, and arrangements are made for them to be met at their arriving station by the person undertaking their aftercare.

All gratuity money due to inmates on their discharge is paid through the person undertaking the aftercare at the rate of 5/- per week, provided they continue to live sober and respectable lives.

The maximum gratuity is [£4:11:3 for a male and £3:8:0 for a female serving 3 year sentence] and in the same ratio for shorter terms. ... In making our arrangements for the aftercare I first interview the inmate and find out his or her intentions, when the cases are willing to be advised by us, we try to get them situations away from their old associations and companions. ... Having fixed the place, we arrange for some person to befriend, supervise and report on the case; this work is now practically all done, either by the After Care Association, of which Mr A.J.S. Maddison, of 32 Charing Cross, London, is the Secretary; or by the National Society for the Prevention of Cruelty to Children, of which Mr. R.J.Parr, of Leicester Square, London, is the Director and Secretary. Mr Maddison, with his agents, is represented in every district to which we discharge, and takes charge of section II. cases. Mr. Parr undertakes the aftercare of section I. cases. A few cases have been discharged to the care for Police Court Missionaries, and a few have been taken up by private families.[72]

The *Inebriates' Reformation and After-care Association* was established in 1898 and in 1906 had 160 agents around the country who would meet discharged inmates to find them lodgings and employment.[73] In addition the agents would control the payment of the gratuities earned by the person whilst in the reformatory, the payment being conditional on good behaviour.

Fleck's management of Brentry ended in 1909 after he oversaw a further public disaster - a mass escape by the men:

early in June [1909] symptoms of unrest were noticed among the men inmates, caused by the expectation of reduced sentences in view of amendments proposed in the Inebriates Acts. This unrest developed later into discontent at the delay in legislation, culminating in a serious disturbance and mutiny on Saturday morning, 3rd July, when no less than 29 men left, but were all captured the same day some distance from the Reformatory.[74]

[The officers] heard what the men said amongst themselves, and among the other inmates. ...Dr Fleck had warned the police to be in readiness, and last Saturday the matter came to a head. A complaint was made about the bread served for breakfast. It so happened that the thundery weather made the yeast 'go off' and that morning it was not so good as usual. Dr Fleck tested the bread, and told the men it was not so nice as usual, but he and the other officers had

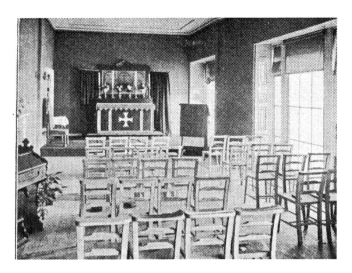

Figure 4.15: The Chapel, converted from old Drawing room in main house.

used it. He also told them he had had a fresh supply of yeast in, and that they could have anything else, except bread. The men did not agree, but apparently marched down to the gate and got away.[75]

[After locking up the other inmates] as many attendants as could be spared set out after the recalcitrants, who had taken the road to Filton. The police were also informed, and Inspector Thompson, of Westbury, with one or two of his men, set off on their bicycles in pursuit. The alarm was also sent to all the surrounding village stations, Hambrook, Stoke Gifford, Thornbury, Patchway, Fishponds, Staple Hill, etc., and police were dispatched in vehicles and on bicycle in all directions.

The fugitives, who were most of them in their shirt sleeves, as soon as they got outside the home armed themselves with tools, sticks and stones, and soon presented a very formidable appearance. Instead of dispersing, as they might have been expected to, they proceeded together down the main road in the direction of Filton, and then striking across the Thornbury highway, proceeded along the road to Patchway and under the railway arch to Hambrook. As they were going through the brickfields some of the searchers overtook them, but they refused to return to the Home, and their strength and numbers forbade arrest. The only thing that could be done was to follow them till reinforcements came.

It was a novel sight to see these recalcitrant fellows strolling at their own pace through the narrow lanes and across fields, stopping here and there to pick a flower. They went quietly enough without opposition, but an attempted check would have brought about disastrous consequences. So the police followed behind pushing their bicycles, carrying them where the ground was too rough to permit of riding or over stiles. …

The mutineers proceeded steadily in the direction of Staple Hill, pausing only and then to demand refreshments at wayside houses. It did not appear polite to refuse them, and when satisfied they went on their way. They had had nearly three hours liberty and had walked many miles when their escort was strengthened suddenly by the arrival of Supt Cooke of Staple Hill with [4 other policemen] and three of the attendants. Supt Cooke at once called on the men to surrender and return to the Home, but they refused, declaring that under no conditions would they be taken back. The superintendent explained that there was only one alternative, and that was they must be locked up in the police station. The reply was that they would rather do that than return to the Home, and this being agreed upon they submitted to being taken by way of Downend to Staple Hill Station, where their presence was a severe tax upon its four cells.[76]

Dr David Fleck tendered his resignation at the next meeting of the Brentry Board on the 26 July 1909. It was accepted and he was asked not to return from his holiday.[77] He left to become medical superintendent of the Burden's Eastern Counties Reformatory at East Harling, before returning to Bristol as the medical officer for Stoke Park. The Board resolved that the next Superintendent of Brentry should not be a medical man, presumably because whilst Fleck had proved 'amiable as an individual and successful as a doctor, [he] failed to secure that amount of firm administration which an Institution of this character must have'.[78] He was succeeded on the 6 October 1909[79] by Commander J. Richard Lay R.N.[Royal Navy] as Superintendent with Ormerod returning to be medical officer. Commander Lay was clearly there to control and immediately entered a dispute about authority between himself and the Chairman of the House Committee, Captain Sampson Way. It was determined that Lay was not subject to Captain Way between the House Committee meetings.[80]

Notes

[1] *Annual report of Inspector 1900*: 1902 (Cd. 811) xii 599

[2] designed by the Site architect, Mr Gabriel (see annual reports)

[3] *Annual report of Inspector 1900*: 1902 (Cd. 811) xii 599 - costs are from the annual reports eg Brentry Certified Inebriate Reformatory: *Annual reports and statements of accounts, for the year ending 31 December 1910*. The evidence of the order of the building is slightly confusing, and suggests that the Inspectors annual reports reflect the state of construction at the time of printing and not necessarily completion during the year of report. What is definite is that the Colony started with the Stables converted for 75 females, then the existing buildings for 30 male beds (Block M) then the Male cottages (N & O - one has '1900' and 'RVH - B' on the eaves), then the Female side was enlarged in 1901 with the female blocks (in June 1901 pamphlet [see below] accommodation is still listed as 75).

[4] Accounts to end 1900, in Minutes of Meetings of 25 March 1901.

[5] This is derived from fact that it is illustrated in the 1901/2 pamphlet.

[6] The Burdens must have lived on site - in 1902 Mr Burden complained that both he and his wife were working 13 hours every day on the site.

[7] *Annual report of Inspector 1900*: 1902 (Cd. 811) xii 599 - costs are from the annual reports eg Brentry Certified Inebriate Reformatory: *Annual reports and statements of accounts, for the year ending 31 December 1910*.The cottages were along Knowle Lane, near Upper Knowle, in the parcel of land enclosed by the Brentry Land

[8] see Resolutions in Board of Management Meetings: Resolution 48, 22 Sept 1899 and 68, 11 December 1899

[9] See accounts of the B.R.I.

[10] Annual report for 1900, 25 March 1901

[11] *Memorandum for the information of Local Authorities wishing to arrange with the Board of Management of the Royal Victoria Homes, for the reception of cases under the above Acts.* - dated June 1901, draft in *BRO*

[12] *Forty Views: The Royal Victoria Homes, Brentry nr Bristol* - not dated but assumed to be 1901 from contents. Copy at *BRO:* 40686/B/BK/1

[13] Brentry June 1901 draft pamphlet (*op cit* – note 11) page 4

[14] For example, *The Times* 12 Jan 1901; *The Birmingham Daily Mail* 27 June 1900; *The Brighton Herald* 26 May 1900; *The Bristol Evening News* 5 January 1901 - all quoted in 1901 pamphlet (note 11)

[15] *Report of the Inspector under the Inebriates Acts ... for 1901*. BPP: 1902 [Cd.1381] **XII** 697. Pages 49-50.

[16] copy states 'presented to both Houses of Parliament' - *GLRO:* CJ1/C1

[17] *Accounts of Expenditure of Wage Earning Women and Girls*. 1911 [Cd.5963] lxxxix 531. It is worth noting that this amount had varied little over 20 years - Charles Booth estimated a similar expenditure for working families in 1889 [Charles Booth *Life and Labour of the People in London. First Series: Poverty 1: East, Central and South London.* [First published 1889] Revised edition London: MacMillan & Co. 1902. (Reprinted New York: Augustus M Kelley,

1969)]

[18] Minutes of Board of Management, 10 December 1900 - report of Finance Committee

[19] Minutes Board of Management, 24 June 1901 page 3

[20] Minutes of Board of Management Meeting 9 December 1901, Finance Committee report - page 4

[21] Warden report, Annual report for 1901

[22] letter by R W Branthwaite, dated 15 April 1901, printed with minutes of Board of Management 29 April 1901

[23] Minutes 25 June 1900

[24] Deputy Warden's Report, in Minutes for 29 April 1901.

[25] Correspondence included in the printed Minutes for 24 June 1901

[26] *BRO:* 40359 /B/3(b) 12 Jan 1903, page 145

[27] *BRO:* 40359/B/3(b) 26 jan 1903 page 150

[28] *BRO:* 40359 /B/3(b) 3 Oct 1902 p118

[29] [29] *Minutes of Evidence taken before the Departmental Committee appointed to inquire into the Operation of the Law relating to Inebriates and to their detention in Reformatories and Retreats.* [Cd.4439]. London: HMSO 1908. Question 23.

[30] see G. Hunt, J. Mellor & J. Turner: 'Wretched, hatless and miserably clad: women and the inebriate reformatories from 1900-1913.' *British Journal of Sociology* 1989 (40): 244-70.

[31] Printed minutes 19 August 1901

[32] Printed minutes 19 August 1901

[33] resolution 64, 9 December 1901

[34] reported in the local papers, but these were said to be inaccurate and an account in included in *BRO:* 40359/B/3(b) minutes p111 for 8 Oct 1902

[35] Printed minutes of special meeting 27 Oct 1902

[36] Foundations had been built by the AGM of 4 Jan 1904, which approved tender of £1165 to build the Kitchen

[37] see correspondence in *BRO* 40359 deposit

[38] Charity Commission Scheme, sealed 17 November 1903 (2983/3, Gloucestershire; Westbury-on-Trym; the Royal Victoria Homes Brentry, near Bristol; A/78,151)

[39] cited in income/expenditure information in Brentry Annual Reports of 1903 and later - 'To transfer to Maintenance account - Amount of deficit as at 31st Dec. 1903: £5171 14s 3d

[40] *Annual report Inspector Reformatories for 1913*: 1914-16 xxiv 37 [Cd 7869]

[41] Printed minutes 23 June 1902

[42] Printed minutes 28 September 1903

[43] see section on RVH.

[44] *BRO:* 40359/B/3(b) Visiting Committee Minute Book No 2. page 24, 21 Dec 1900

[45] *BRO:* 40359/B/3 (b) page 30, 18 Jan 1901; copy of agreement of 6 Jan 1901 in 40359/B/8

[46] BRO 40359 /B/8(a) copy letter from Belfield dated 1 July 1902. To Edward Thomas who was trying to find evidence of agreement.

[47] BRO 40359 /B/8(a) follow up copy letter from Belfield dated 3 August 1902. to Edward Thomas.

[48] *BRO:* 40359/B/8 letter from Parker dated 23 July 1902.

[49] *BRO:* 40359 B/3(b) page 95; 1 Aug 1902 minutes

[50] in *BRO* 40359/B/8

[51] *BRO:* 40359/B/8 letter from Parker dated 23 July 1902.

[52] *BRO:* 40359/B/8 letter dated 2 Aug 1902

[53] *Bristol Daily Mercury* 20 Sept 1902 for notice, *BRO:* 40359 for more details of property for sale

[54] *BRO:* 40359 /B/8 letter of Rev Burden dated 18 Nov 1902

[55] Letter dated 17 March 1902 printed with minutes 24 March 1902

[56] He was also asked by the committee convened to consider his resignation, to accept the post of vice Chairman, and was appointed to this, at the Meeting of 22 June 1903

[57] Deed of 'sale' of Brentry from Edw Thomas and Harold Burden to Trustees of RVH, for the outstanding £1000 on the original mortgage. deposited amongst legal deeds for Brentry held by Bevan Ashfords. This appears to have been done as Mr Thomas when he stopped being the Institution's solicitor, pointed out that he remained personally liable for the repayment of the mortgage (see resolution 57-8 in printed minutes 27 October 1902

[58] *BRO:*40686/NI

[59] the contributions of the *National Institutions* are set out in the Special Meeting of 30 April 1919

[60] See Annual report for 1903, building cost £704. It became part of the Hospital block (Colston)

[61] Printed Minutes Board of Management 5 March 1903

[62] Printed minutes 22 June 1903

[63] letter of resignation dated 20 April 1904, in printed minutes 25 April 1904. Canon Parker's election in Printed minutes 25 July 1904

[64] Printed minutes 26 October 1908

[65] Statement of Edward Cooke, Superintendent at Staple Hill Station, to Chief Constable of Gloucestershire dated 25 June 1906 - *GLRO:* CJ1/C2

[66] *GLRO:* CJ1/C2

[67] *GLRO:* CJ1/C2 letter dated 6 April 1906

[68] *Report of the Inspector on an Outbreak of Enteric Fever at Brentry Inebriate Reformatory* 1908 xii 1141 [Cd.3938]

[69] letter dated 26 June 1908, in printed minutes 27 July 1908

[70] Annual Report for 1905, page 22

[71] *BRO:* 40686/B/BK/2

[72] Dr Flecks report in Brentry Annual Report for 1905, page 18-19

[73] Arthur J. S. Maddison, 'The After-care of Inebriates.' *The British Journal of Inebriety* 1905-6 (3) 40-44.

[74] Printed minutes for 26 July 1909, page 5

[75] *Bristol Times and Mirror* 6 July 1909 p7cd - account of trial

[76] *Bristol Times and Mirror* 5 July 1909 page 9a

[77] resolution 28, in printed minutes meeting 26 July 1909

[78] words of Chairman in Printed minutes 25 April 1910, page 7

[79] Annual Report Brentry 1909

[80] Annual Report Brentry 1909

The Change to Mental Deficiency

Inebriates and Mental Defectives

Soon after the start of the Inebriates Acts came into force it was realised that it was not going to work as intended. Many rebelled and it was found that overall 'about 10 to 15 per cent were too unmanageable to retain in certified reformatories under surroundings so desirably light and unprison-like.'[1] In addition in 1905 the published legal commentary for magistrates was that to be classified as a 'habitual drunkard', one had to be incapable of managing ones affairs *when sober* as well as when drunk.[2] The result was that most being sent to reformatories after this date were classifiable as 'mental defectives' and had an even lower success rate.

Even before this legal comentary there already was a view that many inebriates were feeble-minded, if only to justify why reformatories were not working. This is highlighted in the considerations of the Royal Commission on the Care and Control of the Feeble-minded who met from 1904 to 1908. The Rev. Burden, as a 'manager of inebriate reformatories', was appointed to the Commission. This was in part as he was a friend of several of the high officials of the Home Office and was seen as a useful man in generating accommodation where needed. But it was also because it was thought initially that inebriacy should be included within the terms of feeble-minded. The Commission heard evidence on this matter in its early meetings.

Whilst they were hearing evidence Robert Branthwaite expressed his opinion as inspector of inebriate reformatories.

> The more experience we have in the detention of committed inebriates the more we are finding close relationship to the condition which ordinarily apply to the detention of lunatics. Inebriate reformatories are little other than modified asylums for the detention of mentally defective persons, and the end of each year finds us more closely approximating the routine of our institutions to the routine of lunatic asylums. All our arrangements as to discipline, punishments, associated and solitary feeding, sleeping, exercise, recreation and work, are controlled and regulated by individual mental and physical indications.[3]

In his annual report for 1905 he wrote that mental defect was a cause of inebriacy and also a cause of the failure of some to respond to the 'therapy' of the reformatories. His report has a large section highlighting the issue of mental defect in inebriates, with photographs to illustrate the features of defectives.[4] He estimated that of the 1873 people admitted to reformatories, 14.5% had been "very defective - Imbeciles, degenerates and epileptics" and 45.7% "Defective - eccentric, silly, dull, senile, or subject to paroxysms of ungovernable temper". He justified this classification with the moral certainty that such things as behaviour after years of drinking indicated congenital weaknesses:

> Our present object, however, is merely to justify the assertion that mental incompetence, stopping short of insanity, holds a prominent position in the causation of habitual drunkenness, and complete irresponsibility for drunkenness may result therefrom....
> Certain peculiarities in cranial conformation, general physique, and conduct, have long been recognised as evidences of congenital defect. Nearly all the 1,128 cases included in the defective sections of our table have given evidence of possessing some of these characteristic peculiarities, and it is morally certain that the large majority of them started life handicapped by weakness....
> The photographs ... illustrate in a convincing manner the presence of defect, mostly congenital; even the untrained eye should meet with no difficulty in recognising the signs in most of them.[5]

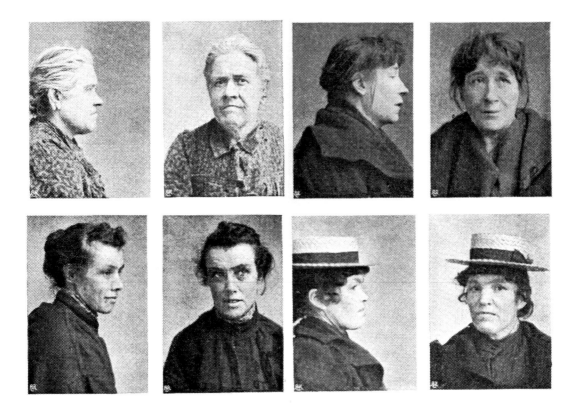

Figure 5.1: Inebriate women showing 'the presence of defect'

His photographs (four are shown in Figure 5.1) may well have come from Brentry, though no photographs remain in its records. They are a telling image of the typical ladies admitted to Brentry at the time. In this period mental deficiency, like many other social conditions, was diagnosed as much by appearance as by performance. Branthwaite was therefore not unusual in discussing the stigmata of mental deficiency.

Dr David Fleck, the medical superintendent for Brentry echoed Branthwaite's views when he gave evidence to the Royal Commission on the Care and Control of the Feeble Minded:

> Although ... physical peculiarities are not so evident amongst inebriates as they are amongst idiots and imbeciles, still an examination of our cases shows in less degree a tendency to similar deformities. This I have convinced myself is a very strong indication that many of the cases sent to me for care and treatment belong to the same class of defectives. ... In the absence of any exact standard for our guidance it is exceedingly difficult to draw hard and fast lines between those of defective mental condition and those of fair capacity; but as a rule no difficulty arises in discriminating between sound and unsound.
> Seven hundred and seventy-one cases have been committed to Brentry since [its opening] ...In my opinion about 30 per cent may be considered of fair mental capacity ... With consideration to the remaining 70 per cent I cannot conceive the possibility of their ever acquiring sufficient self-control to be able to keep from drunkenness and support themselves. ... In my opinion, however, nearly all these cases have started life handicapped, and have added to the original injury by their irregular habits....
> Of this number [the 70%] a small percentage has been found to be certifiably insane, and these have accordingly been sent to lunatic asylums for special treatment. ... A further small percentage has been composed of epileptics requiring constant supervision and permanent control. ... [It is difficult to describe] the mental condition of the balance of our defectives ... Generally speaking they are restless, excitable, wanting in reasoning power, unable to concentrate or keep to fixed ideas, impulsive in the extreme and suspicious to

an extent almost amounting to delusion; refinements are masked, and the baser passions prevail, lying is common, and a tendency to deceive is always present. Profanity, vile language and uncontrolled passion become evident on the least provocation; morbid sexual excitement, irregularity and perversion are not uncommon....

The results of our treatment on those of fair mental capacity are very encouraging, and I think satisfactory. Some of our inmates showing mental defect in milder form improve under treatment and are, therefore, possibly reformable, but so far as the majority of our defectives are concerned there is little hope of reformation, the effort comes too late; they are, in my opinion, cases for an indeterminate sentence, or in other words they should be committed for permanent control, there being suitable provision for periodical revision of the sentence as the condition of each case warrants.[6]

The Royal Commission on the Care and Control of the Feeble-Minded issued their report in 1908. They decided that the care of inebriates did not fall within their remit. They favoured caring for 'mental defectives' in specially designed residential homes or colonies. They recommended residential care if the person could not be adequately supervised in the community.They did not require permanent care but were keen for the long term protection of these people. The Rev. Burden added his own memorandum to the main recommendations:

I am in complete agreement with the Report as a whole. But I should like to give prominence to the need for economy in and strict Governmental control over the establishment of institutions for the reception of mentally defective persons.
The cost of establishment of institutions for mentally defective persons not requiring special medical treatment should not cost the ratepayer anything approaching the amount expended on present day-asylums. The erection of institutions at an expenditure involving the payment of 8s to 10s per bed per week for interest, repayment of loans, and such-like charges alone should, I am convinced, be wholly a thing of the past.
I am of opinion that the cost of building an institution for the mentally defective (other than for "persons of unsound mind") should never exceed £150 a bed, and for many of the classes of the mentally defective suitable provision can be made at a cost not exceeding £100 a bed.[7]

His dealings over inebriates with the Home Office and Local Authorities had clearly reinforced for him that economy and value-for-money were very important, just as they still are.

Though the Royal Commission reported in 1908 the new Liberal Government was too busy to act upon its recommendations. It was finally stung into action after the Eugenics Society and others drafted their own 'Feeble-Minded Control Bill' and persuaded some MPs to introduce it into parliament in 1912. This failed, but as a result the Government produced a modified version of this bill and it was passed as the Mental Deficiency Act in 1913.[8]

Apart from "Idiots" and "Imbeciles", the Act defined the following classes of persons who were mentally defective:

(c) Feeble-minded persons; that is to say, persons in whose case there exists from birth or from an early age mental defectiveness not amounting to imbecility, yet so pronounced that they require care, supervision, and control for their own protection or for the protection of others, or, in the case of children, that they by reason of such defectiveness appear to be permanently incapable of receiving proper benefit from the instruction in ordinary schools;
(d) Moral Imbeciles; that is to say, persons who from an early age display some permanent mental defect coupled with strong vicious or criminal propensities on which punishment has had little or no deterrent effect.

These definitions do not include any statement about defective intelligence, or of poor performance on formal intelligence tests. This was because intelligence testing was still in its infancy and as there was a strong feeling that mental defectiveness was a defect in social functioning rather than intellectual functioning. For example the important medical writer Tredgold wrote that the best test of mental defectiveness was the ability to live independently, and not any formal intelligence test. As a result many of the people detained as being a mental defective (for example feeble minded) were of normal intelligence. Indeed one of the problems in many mental defective colonies was that the inmates could be more intelligent than the nurses.

The definition of 'moral defective' could be applied to paedophiles or single mothers, as well as to people later called 'psychopaths'. Most of those so labelled were of normal intelligence.

Almost anyone who needed 'control' could be called 'feeble-minded'. Some of the specific groups of people are set out in the list of when a mentally defective person could be placed under guardianship or in an institution for mental defectives:[9]

At the instance of his parent or guardian:

- If he was an idiot or imbecile,
- If he was feeble-minded, or a moral Imbecile, and still a child (under 21).

By legal authorities:

- If he was found neglected, abandoned, without visible means of support, or if cruelly treated.
- Or if convicted of a criminal offence, or if as a child he was liable to be ordered to be sent to an industrial school [Borstal].
- Or if he was already in prison, in an industrial school, in an inebriate reformatory or in a lunatic asylum.
- Or if he was a habitual drunkard within the meaning of the Inebriates Acts.
- Or if she was in receipt of poor relief at the time of being pregnant with, or giving birth to, an illegitimate child.
- Or if he was aged less than 17 and about to leave a special [education] class, and where the local education authority 'are of the opinion that it would be to their benefit that they be' so placed.

The orders for detention were to last initially only one year, but could be renewed for the remainder of the person's life so long as the order was 'required in his interests' in the view of the staff.[10]

This new Mental Deficiency Act clearly included powers over people previously dealt with under the Inebriates Acts, but was more powerful in enabling life-long placement in institutions rather than only a maximum of 3 years.

The Collapse of the Inebriate Acts

The increasing frustration with the low rates of success with inebriates came to a head in 1906 when the Treasury cut its grant for cases in reformatories, on the grounds that the costs of the Rev. Burden's *National Institutions* was less than the Treasury grant. London County Council responded by cancelling its contracts with the *National Institutions* and sending only the more obviously treatable cases to reformatories. The number of persons admitted nationally had been consistently rising since 1899 but now almost halved from 493 in 1907 to 262 in 1908. It recovered slightly afterwards but admissions ran at a steady 300 a year until 1913.[11] The system was now overprovided. In 1910 the Rev Burden complained to the Home Office that his new contract with the London County Council was 'most unsatisfactory' as they were not sending enough cases, but that he had had to sign it. He warned that:

> It is I fear very obvious that unless the number of cases committed is <u>greatly</u> increased, it will be hopeless for me to attempt to carry on more than one of our Reformatories. I am closing Lewes next week, and I see no alternative to closing Ackworth, Chesterfield, and Horfield as soon as I can conveniently do so. I hope to continue to use the East Harling premises as an Inebriate Reformatory, but unless the committals are sufficiently numerous it will be impossible to do so indefinitely.[12]

Though the Royal Commission on the Poor Laws advocated early intervention and committal,[13] the magistrates continued to turn against the use of the inebriate acts. A survey of the magistrates of London in March 1910 gave the inebriate reformatories no hope of recovery:

> Mr Garrett: Has long ceased to look upon Inebriate Homes as Reformatories and merely uses them as places of detention for women who are an intolerable nuisance. All such cases as have been before him for some time past have already been in Inebriate Homes.
> Mr Fordham: Cases which he considers fit for treatment in Reformatory seldom come before him. Doubts usefulness of treatment but sends cases at all likely to benefit. Finds that the threat to send to Reformatory is effective.
> Mr Hutton: … Remarks on strangeness of authorities devoting almost exclusive attention to women who are as a rule practically irreformable whereas men are less difficult subjects for treatment.
> Mr Mead: Does not intend to send any more cases to Inebriate Reformatories. Every single case committed has returned and been convicted again of drunkenness. Perhaps remedy of Reformatory treatment is not applied soon enough by magistrates but the fault is rather in the restricted definition of "habitual drunkard". Has long felt that workhouses sufficient substitutes for "these expensive institutions", viz Inebriate Reformatories.[14]

A failed attempt was made to resurrect the reformatories with new legislation in 1912, but at this time people expected many of the inebriates to be dealt with under the new Mental Deficiency Act. Many campaigners preferred the indefinite confinement authorised by the Mental Deficiency Act to the fixed maximum of three years under the Inebriacy Acts, and so stopped pressing for a new Inebriacy law.

In 1913 the London County Council carried a resolution to close its inebriate reformatory, Farmfield. The Home Office was aghast.

> If this resolution is carried out, and Mr Burden closes most of his Reformatories, the work will practically come to an end. This would mean a deplorable waste of money and labour. A certain proportion of the inebriates might be dealt with under the Mental Deficiency Act, but for the rest we should lose a piece of machinery which is not only beneficial to many inebriates, but also useful for the public.[15]

The London County Council promised to reconsider its decision if a new inebriate bill was passed during 1914, but the Government said it could not do this, though it asked the Treasury to carry on paying higher rates of subsidy to the reformatories to postpone the Farmfield decision.[16]

Brentry Certified Institution

Though the demand for places in Inebriate Reformatories fell from 1908 onwards it almost totally collapsed in the war when the sale of alcohol was restricted and convictions for drunkenness dramatically reduced. All the reformatories run by the *National Institutions* closed in turn, often to temporarily become mental deficiency colonies. Because the *National Institutions* sent their cases to Brentry as they closed its inmate numbers remained high at over 200 until 1915. This still meant that by 1910 there were many vacant beds and a continuing revenue deficit despite all attempts to correct it. Though in 1911, a small ward for sick men was opened[17] no other planned developments were carried out for some time.

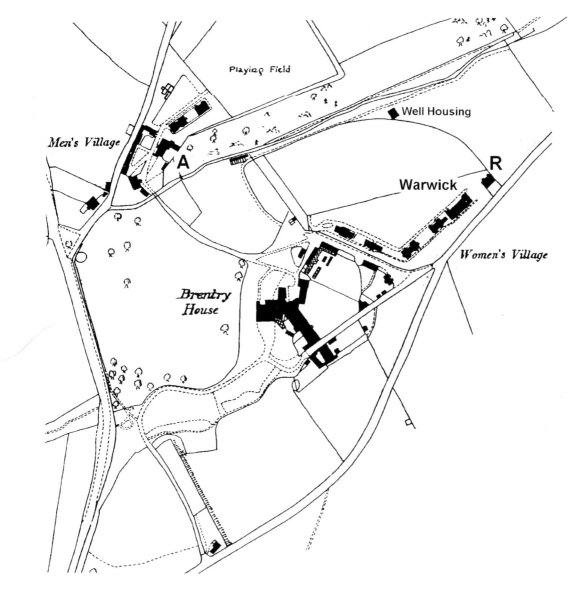

Figure 5.2: Brentry in 1922 – A is the 1907 ward, R is the women's receiving house

The final transfer of inebriates from other institutions came in November 1915 when the London County Council closed its reformatory at Farmfield and transferred the 45 female inmates to Brentry[18] before it converted Farmfield to being a mental deficiency colony. As well as having been the first licensed Inebriate Reformatory in England Brentry became the last, struggling with the staff shortages generated by the war.

At the end of 1915, the future of Brentry as an Inebriate Reformatory was bleak. After a few marginally good quarters (in part due to low staffing levels due to the war) it was again running in deficit and had an accumulated debt of £3000 of expenditure over income. There were no other reformatories to empty into it and admissions were at an all time low despite it being the only inebriate reformatory in England. As inebriates could only be confined for up to three years it was clear that the institution would be virtually empty by the end of 1918.

The Board decided to set up a committee to look at Brentry's future as a reformatory.[19] In March 1916 it was decided to ask councils to permit an application to the Charity Commission for a change in the purposes of Brentry to also accept mental defectives. This was agreed and on 16 December 1916 the Charity Commission approved a new scheme permitting this.[20] The Board of Control certified part of the lower colony as a colony for 125 male adult mental defectives[21] and made very encouraging noises:

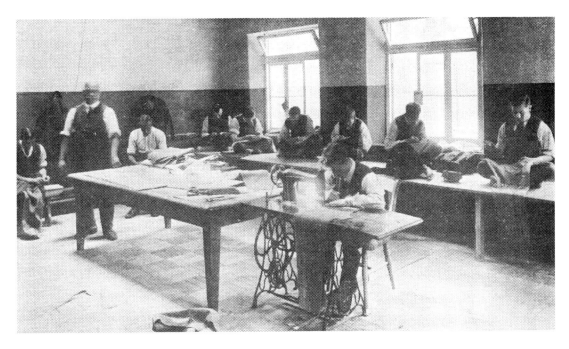

Figure 5.3: Tailoring in the new workshop.

one part of the Men's Village certified... The buildings erected on the cottage system therefore favouring classification are especially suitable for housing Male Defectives. Successful development of enterprise has been delayed by staff difficulties owing to the war: recently action by the Managers, however, appears likely to ensure the success of the undertaking. Accommodation for adult Male Defectives is in great demand and an Institution on the Brentry lines should prove valuable to the work.[22]

The first 11 new inmates were admitted in June 1917[23] to the lower village. The committee initially wished to certify the women village for female Mental Defectives.[24] Within a year they were told that both villages had to be used for men in order to obtain an adequate variety of buildings to enable classification of inmates[25] and in 1919 the licence was increased by a further 105 so that the site was licensed for 230 Adult Male Mental Defectives.[26] There was no licence for the admission of children because the Board of Education was against feeble-minded children being admitted to inebriate reformatories.[27]

This transfer from being an inebriate reformatory to a colony for adult male mental defectives was not unique to Brentry. Farmfield transferred from being a female inebriate reformatory to a mental deficiency colony for adult males. Cattal (or Whixley) in Yorkshire made the same transition shortly after Farmfield.[28] The Langho reformatory in Lancashire probably also did so. Only the Midland reformatory is known to have changed from being a reformatory for female inebriates to being a colony for female mental defectives when the *National Institutions*, now renamed the *National Institutions for Persons Requiring Care and Control [NIPRCC]*, changed it to Whittington Hall Colony. This initial demand for beds for male mental defectives contrasts strongly with the demand for female inebriate beds. It probably was because the male mental defectives were less likely to have dependants than the inebriate men and were more likely than females to be seen as a nuisance who were difficult to control in the existing institutions of care.

At the same time as the growth of the inmate population of male mental defectives at Brentry there was a rapid run down of the number of Inebriates. By the end of 1917 there were only 11 men and 49 women left. At this time the Rev Burden as secretary and Dr Branthwaite as inspector suggested that to admit more mental defectives the inebriate women should be moved from the upper village to the old stables and main building. Sir Henry Mather-Jackson resisted the idea saying the buildings were too gloomy and would give too poor a result. His resistance made the Home Office comment that 'Sir Henry Jackson' was 'an old gentleman who has been Chairman of Brentry since its foundation and is extremely interested in the place',[29] implying that though a good man he was out of touch with modern realities and practice. In January 1918 the Brentry Committee wrote to the Home Secretary, stating that there were now only 8 male inebriates in the colony and soon would be only 6. They asked if the Secretary of State felt the expenditure justified and 'if he would authorise the discharge of the six cases referred to'.[30] He agreed but by the end of the year there remained one man as well as 18 women. The last man left soon afterwards and in 1920, when an application was made to admit a male inebriate the Home Office stated that there was now no reformatory accommodation in the country to take Male Inebriates.[31] The final 6 ladies finally moved into the stable wing of the main administration block. The last admission of an inebriate was admission Number 957, a woman admitted on 11 March 1921. The last two inmates were discharged on the 31 October 1921,[32] the day the licence for inebriates was formally surrendered. The Inebriate Acts remained in force but with no practical usefulness until they were repealed in the 1970s.

The changeover to Mental Deficiency did not solve Brentry's financial difficulties. Filling vacancies was slow and compounded by the war causing staffing and building problems. Yet again most of the placements came from the *NIPRCC*. There was a minimum of 60 vacancies a year until 1920 when it again reached 220 occupants. In addition to these revenue losses Brentry had to undertake a few capital projects to enable the change to Mental Defectives and support the 47 staff listed in July 1917.[33] The consequence was a period of large deficits.[34]

In January 1917 the Contributing Councils were again asked to bail out the Colony, with a further £10 per reserved bed.[35] Most councils agreed and £2000 working capital was obtained. However this did not change the revenue deficits and in July 1918 the Finance Committee recommended that an emergency committee be constituted to examine how to resolve the crisis.[36]

At this time there seems to have been covert and rival pressure from the Burdens' *NIPRCC* and from Bristol City Council to acquire Brentry. Mr Burden was in a strong position being both a member of the Emergency Committee and a financial help to Brentry. A conference on the 17 February, attended mainly by people from Bristol, suggested that no action should occur for 3 months (presumably so they could carry out more negotiations) but the Chairman pointed out that the enterprise could not clearly survive its debts for this time:

> the Bank's friendly attitude towards us has been very largely due to the influence of Mr Burden who is known to the manager as a person of substance and I fancy that it is largely owing to this that we have been able to get along at all.[37]

He pointed out that with the debts

> a very critical position may easily arise at any time, especially if Mr Burden were to take umbrage at the unwillingness of the Board to accept the terms offered by the Incorporation, despite his assurances that he is anxious to help us out of our difficulties.

And he recommended action. The result was a special meeting on the 26 February 1919, when it was suggested that either

a) Brentry be closed and the site sold;

b) the Contributing Councils agree run it directly as a co-operative, and pay whatever it cost to run

or (c) it be transferred to a body such as the Burdens' *Incorporation of National Institutions for Persons Requiring Care and Control* [*Inc.NIPRCC*](which was the name of the company that ran the colonies owned by the *NIPRCC*).

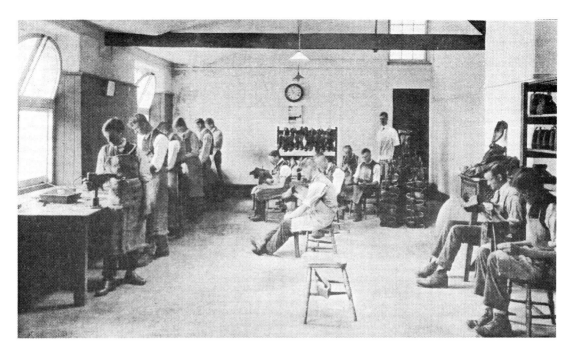

Figure 5.4: Bootmaking in new workshop

It was agreed that Brentry should not be transferred to the *Inc.NIPRCC*, and that some of the councils explore taking it over. The meeting was adjourned to the 30 April 1919.

The Chairman, wrote to the Rev Burden after this, repudiating part of the minutes the Rev. Burden had taken of the meeting and attacking his role in the decisions:

> With regard to the last paragraph "The Incorporation if willing to submit a Scheme to do so also before that date, the two schemes to be considered together" are your words and not mine, but as you represent the Incorporation tho' I confess I did not understand you then to make this qualification I must now accept it. I am quite at a loss to understand what the real attitude of the Incorporation is and at no two meetings I have had with you since the idea of a change began to be considered have the intentions of the Incorporation appeared to be the same. When I first broached the subject you promised to see the Chairman and let me have his views, then later on you said there would be a meeting of your Council and you bring it before them, then you sent me the letter which I, and others thought was an offer, then came your repudiation of it as such at the meeting and now comes the draft report.[38]

He sent a copy of this to the Clerk of the Gloucestershire Mental Deficiency Committee, Mr Gardom, with the accompanying explanatory letter:

> I was sorry not to be able to support your views on Wednesday, but - I know my man. I send you a copy of a letter I have written to him today. you will think it perhaps a little strong, but he is quite pachydermous. It is never possible to pin him to anything and you saw it for yourself on Wednesday. It has been well said that there are "men women and parsons", and there never was better proof of it than in this case. It has always been so, and tho' I must admit it is strange that the other Institutions under him are a success he has never attempted to make this go well. Whether it has been all along his wish to "wreck it" and come in on salvage terms or not I do not know, but I am quite satisfied no joint management will work. I hope you and Bristol will knock up something. If you do not and the Incorporation do not take it over there can be no alternative to closing and selling the Property.
> I write for you eyes alone - I have suffered much at the hands of this person!!![39]

At the meeting on 30 April 1919[40] a consortium of Bristol, Somerset and Bath offered to take Brentry over for 25% of the outlay, as they needed a mental deficiency colony. The councils on the Board of Management were reluctant to give up a colony that was a potential source of beds for their local needs, and welcomed the rival offer of Mr Burden. He asked if the *Inc.NIPRCC* could purchase the institution, which was again rejected but his alternative that the *Inc.NIPRCC* offered a cash loan for a formal place on the Board of Management was accepted, despite all of Mather-Jackson's private reservations about joint management. The result was a loan of £6400 by the *Inc.NIPRCC*, and the alterations to the premises which enabled the Board of Control to increase the licence by 105 to 230 male mental defectives. The *Inc.NIPRCC* entered into a written agreement with the Brentry Management Committee for mutual interchange and admission of cases and the *Inc.NIPRCC* arranged the direct admission or transfer of 74 men to Brentry. By March 1920 the books balanced for the first time in five years.[41]

As part of the new Board arrangements the management was remodeled on that of the *Inc.NIPRCC*. One General Committee replaced all the existing sub-committees (Finance, Buildings and General Purposes).[42] Similarly the rules of the *Inc.NIPRCC* were adopted for Brentry.[43] Brentry now operated almost as another branch of the *Inc.NIPRCC* with admissions controlled by the *Inc.NIPRCC* central offices and the staff governed by *Inc.NIPRCC* rules. However the managing councils still had admitting rights and rights to lower fees, and they also determined the day-to-day policies and staff employed at the colony. The Charity Commissioner were asked to approve the revised scheme and did so on 3 January 1922 when they changed the name of *Brentry Certified Institution and Inebriate Reformatory* to *Brentry Certified Institution,*[44] recognising the demise of the reformatory.

The change in inmates was associated with a change in the superintendent. Commander Lay had been called up for service during the war but tried to give some support from his port base in England[45]. The Home Office was very unhappy with this and wrote to his Admiral:

> May I trouble you for some information on the position of Commander Lay, who is at present employed as a Transport Officer and is working, I believe, at Southampton.
> Commander Lay is Superintendent of Brentry Inebriate Reformatory a large Institution under voluntary management for men and women ... the present arrangement is that the men's part of the Reformatory is left in charge of an Assistant Superintendent, a man who is only suitable for a subordinate post, and the women's part is left in charge of the Matron. Commander Lay visits once a week and is in frequent telephone contact.
> We have received unsatisfactory reports in the present condition of the Institution and it appears to use essential that a man of suitable qualifications should be placed in charge. [We beg to inquire] whether Commander Lay can be released from his Admiralty work whether now or in the near future.?[46]

He was not released. Though Commander Lay offered the prospect of an imminent transfer to Avonmouth and though the reformatory was found to be in a reasonable state on a surprise inspection,[47] he was obliged to resign on 27 June 1918.[48] He was replaced by Mr Thomas R. Lambert and his wife who started work as Superintendent and Matron on 1 July. Mr Lambert came 'from a well-managed public Institution of a somewhat similar character'.[49] Rather unfortunately, Mrs Lambert was ill and was unable to start work as Matron for a short time. Dr Ormerod remained as Medical Officer.

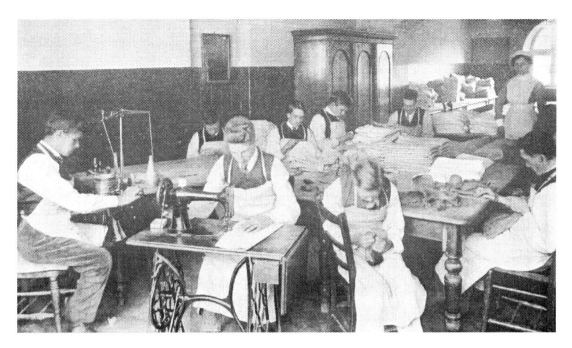

Figure 5.5: Sewing in the new workshop

The first attempts to care for 'mental defectives'

Brentry was a unique institution in being operated by a consortium of councils and the *Inc.NIPRCC*. For most of the councils it provided a few beds for male inmates at some distance from their home area. They would not have had any real commitment to the place and would have found it useful for men not wanted in local institutions. Trouble was inevitable.

In July 1921 a Gloucestershire official visited Brentry to review the 'mental defectives' and left very dissatisfied. She reported to the Gloucestershire Mental Deficiency Committee that the patients were dejected, miserable and untidily clothed.[50] As a result the Clerk to the Committee and its medical advisor made an unannounced visit. Mr Lambert was away on holiday so an attendant showed them around. They saw the men felling trees and cleaning the drive. They saw the patients having tea in the lower village - 115 standing to say the Lords prayer, then eating bread (3-4" thick) with a small square of marge on top and a mug of tea. They were told that the Lower Village was the place for criminal and rough cases and that unruly patients from the Upper Village were sent there 'for long and short periods'. They concluded that[51]

> 1) The Institution is as well managed as it can under existing conditions;
> 2) The establishment has a general air of roughness;
> 3) Absconding is far too common;
> 4) The patients general appearance was clean and healthy.

The Clerk Mr Gardom separately noted that the 'lads with criminal propensities' should not be at Brentry but in a State or similar Institution. They were a bad influence and

> It is stated to be practically impossible for the staff at Brentry to prevent absconding and the inhabitants in the neighbourhood of the Institution have complained of offences committed by Inmates of this Class.

Later a group from West Ham visited and were generally satisfied, noting that the unoccupied patients were of too 'low type' to be able to be occupied. They did however comment that:

> This Institution seems to be used as a dumping ground for all those cases that there does not appear to be suitable places for. There are about 12 cases, all of which show criminal tendencies, who are demoralising the whole of the others

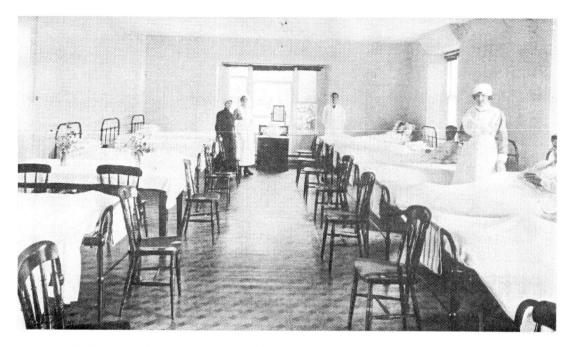

Figure 5.6: The new hospital sick ward in the main building.

> there, and we are of opinion that such cases should be transferred to a suitable Institution, such as the Rampton Institution.
> We feel the Superintendent is working under a hopeless handicap while such cases remain, and that more Hospital accommodation should be provided at once.[52]

Yet again Brenty was being sent the 'wrong type' of person, only they were now called mental defectives and not inebriates.

The problem of absconding is repeatedly remarked on for many years, and the local parish council once publicly complained about the frequent escapes.[53]

The romance behind one of these escapes is revealed in May 1923 in a letter from the Superintendent to the Board of Control requesting the removal of two men to Rampton:

> Adjoining the Lower Village grounds there is a Market Garden where two young women are employed ... they have attracted the attention of these two inmates and surreptitiously communications have passed between them. The inmates broke bounds during the evening of the 25 April and our Officers discovered them in a thickly covered wood two or three miles away [Berwick Woods] in the company of the women. Owing to the darkness they spent the night there and were rounded up in the early hours next morning and brought back to the Institution. I cautioned them and kept them in bed for three days to prevent a recurrence. This morning I intercepted [this] letter written ... to one of the women ... and the women will insist on walking along the public highway for the same purpose....[54]

> My Darling Annie,
>   I am writing this few lines to you hoping you are quite well as it leaves me. I have had 3 days bred and water and you can bet I am starving. Well dear I hope you have not done with me if you have I am going to run away again so for God sacke dont say you have. I hope you have not got in to any trubbul over me. I can not get enney sleep over you dear I hope you are not going out with that Frank I dont think you are dear because I trust you wile I am in hear and I want you to trust me do you think you could.
> By the way dear did you send me enney fags up if you did I got them all write

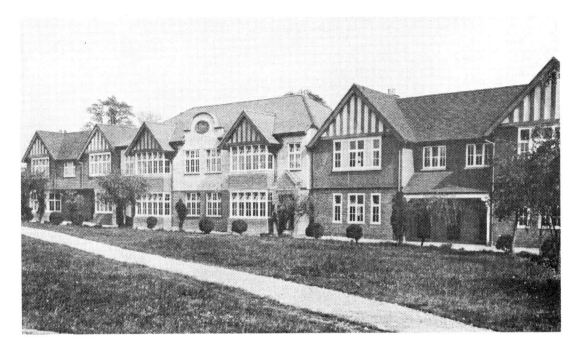

Figure 5.7: The new super ward. 'B' Block

thank you. Well dear I think this is all for this time so good bye my God bless you
& Jean always.
Frome your
　　　unhapey Boy
　　　　　Len
Write back to me dear as soon as you can.
Dear the Officers are going to send the rings back to you they wont let us have
them.

The Board of Control Inspector visited on the 5 May 1922 and wrote a critical report. Dr Gill criticised the Hospital block and said separate accommodation was needed for Tubercular cases. He criticised the lack of night attendants for the hospital, dreary day rooms and poor lavatories (which irritated the committee as the Board of Control had approved all the past designs and as Dr Gill did not allow for the inmates blocking up the toilets with foreign objects). He criticised the lack of occupation; the large proportion of inmates 'addicted to degrading habits, in some cases of a very gross type' and the lack of staff employed to train the 'boys'. He noted that in 13 months twenty patients had absconded on 24 occasions. This report reveals that for the 233 patients (four of whom were missing without leave) there was a head attendant with 10-11 attendants on duty at any time, a cook, mason, basket maker, carpenter, painter, 2 engineers and 4 farm/garden hands. There was only one night staff for each village. Apart from the matron the only women were the laundress and seamstress. None of the attendants were resident, unlike many asylums.

The Board of Control circulated the report to the Contributing Councils before meeting with the Brentry Chairman to discuss it.[55] A fresh building programme was agreed. During 1922 a Boot-maker Instructor and a Tailor Instructor were employed.[56] The Stables vacated by the last inebriates was converted into a new set of workshops, opened in September 1923 containing the Tailors (Figure 5.3), Bootmaking (Figure 5.4), basket making, mat making, barbers and a classroom.[57] There was also a sewing room (Figure 5.5). It was originally planned to convert the stables wing into a new hospital, but instead the 3 storey annex to the main building was converted to a new hospital (Figure 5.6) and opened in March 1924.[58] The feeble and epileptic patients were moved to the old hospital (later called Dickens block).[59]

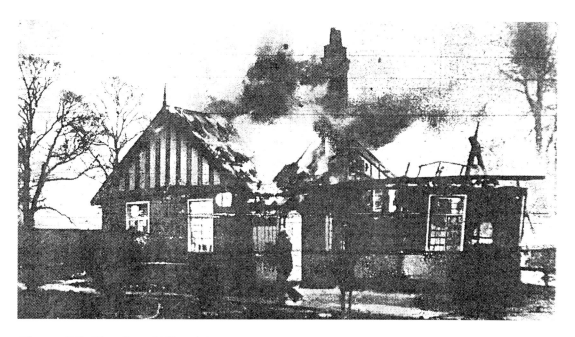

Figure 5.8: The fire at Warwick

The use of the Colony for Mental Defectives, led to changes in the buildings as well as staff. The fees charged for 'Mental Defectives' was less than that for Inebriates. Dr Branthwaite (now a commissioner on the Board of Control and a 'good friend' of Brentry as well as of Mr Burden) recommended that to be financially successful they had to build a further 80 beds as cheaply as possible.[60] He repeated this advice in a more formal report as a Board of Control Inspector to ensure it was widely read.[61] To provide more beds the original two cottage blocks in the top village were joined up (Figure 5.7). This was initially planned to create 48 extra beds as well as merging the two cottages into a single ward to reduce staffing, running a single ward that came to eventually contain a monstrous 118 beds.

Then on Wednesday 11 March 1925 'Warwick' block burnt down (Figure 5.8). The two-storey temporary building built in 1903[62] provided 15 beds along with day-space and a dining room for the adjacent blocks and an officers' mess. Fortunately though 40 patients were in the building at the time no lives were lost. The officers' mess was rebuilt onto the old infirmary (Top village, block A in Figure 6.5) at the end furthest from the Village Hall. Due to the loss of patient facilities, the new large combined ward opened in March 1926 with eight fewer extra beds. The old female receiving house was pressed into use as a further dormitory with 11 beds.

Immediately after the fire it was planned to replace Warwick with a block for 100 inmates but 'C', the block that was opened on the site on Warwick on 27 July 1927[63] (Figure 5.9) contained only 60 beds and a private ward. It cost £5850, funded by the insurance on the old Warwick and a £4000 donation by Gloucestershire to buy 40 of the beds to be built. By means of these enlargements, Brentry held 347 men by 1928.

In the middle of the building work though the Board of Control pressed the Management Board at Brentry to sell it to Bristol and other local councils, as previously proposed. In 1925 they had a meeting with the management committee and said that mental defectives should be in institutions readily accessible to their relatives.[64] This was to no avail and Bristol had to continue to look for another Mental Deficiency Colony whilst using the Stapleton Workhouse as a temporary solution. Bristol eventually built Hortham Colony at Almondsbury in 1933. Hortham claimed it was the first colony built from scratch on a green field site under the 1913 Mental Deficiency Act.

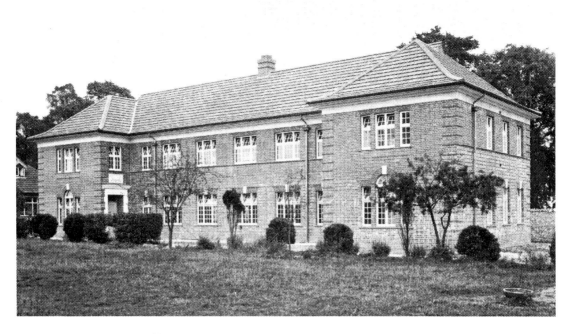

Figure 5.9: The new 'C' block.

During the following period several councils opted out of Brentry as they developed more local facilities. In 1928 Gloucestershire acquired the interests of Hertfordshire to become the biggest council with 47 reserved beds. Monmouthshire acquired the interests of Somerset, Bristol, and Bath and with an extra £1000 gained rights to 46 beds. Reading bought out Birkenhead's interests to attain rights to 14 beds[65] whilst Birmingham gained rights to 20 beds. The management was becoming more committed to the place, as Brentry became a major colony for both Gloucestershire and Monmouthshire.

The Board of Control decided that matters had improved when they visited in January 1928[66] but they were still a long way from being perfect. They found that three patients had absconded and that the lower village was still used for the more troublesome cases, though some of the more amenable cases were placed there as well due to lack of space. The lower village had to eat cold puddings because its dining hall was so far from the central kitchen. The inmates of its B block had no chairs to sit on. The upper village had inadequate day-space and was overcrowded. The 'very important part of training', physical drill, was given inadequate attention and none of the 15 attendants were trained. 'Many are quite interested in their work, but some do not appear to appreciate that they are dealing with undeveloped minds in adult bodies and address their charges in none too kind a tone.' They recommended that some of the staff be sent for training. They also noted that the case books showed little detail apart from admission detail and 'is not a record of progress.' The Colony was still operating as a custodial institution and was struggling. Though the statements made about good colonies were rather idealistic (See Appendix 4) it was clear that Brentry still needed radical reform.

Notes

[1] *Minutes of Evidence taken before the Departmental Committee appointed to inquire into the Operation of the Law relating to Inebriates and to their detention in Reformatories and Retreats.* [Cd.4439]. London: HMSO 1908. Question 23.

[2] *Minutes of Evidence taken before the Departmental Committee ...* [Cd.4439] page 17.

[3] *PRO*: HO45/10052/A63072 /5; 14 Dec 1907.

[4] *Annual report of the Inspector of Reformatories for 1905.* BPP: 1906[Cd.3246]xvi 1.

[5] *Annual report of the Inspector of Reformatories for 1905.* BPP: 1906[Cd.3246]xvi 1. Pages 10-11.

[6] *Report of the Royal Commission on the Care and Control of the Feeble Minded*, Vol 5 (1908 xxxviii 1 [Cd.4219]) pages 242-3: Appendix 12j - Statement by David Fleck Esq. M.B.

[7] *Report ...* Vol 8: [Cd.4202] 1908 xxxix 159: page 511

[8] *An Act to make further and better provision for the care of Feeble-minded and other Mentally Defective Persons and to amend the Lunacy Acts.* 3 & 4 Geo.5, Ch. 28. *Mental Deficiency Act 1913*

[9] Mental Deficiency Act 1913, section 2 and 3.

[10] Mental Deficiency Act 1913, section 11.

[11] See various annual *Report of the Inspector under the Inebriates Acts...* Particularly report for 1912.

[12] *PRO*: HO45/10533-151107/57 dated 3 January 1910.

[13] *Report of the Royal Commission on the Poor Laws and relief of distress.* 1909 [Cd.4499] Part 8 Chapter 7.

[14] PRO: HO45/10533-151107/62 dated 22 March 1910

[15] PRO: HO45/10533-151107/85 dated 8 August 1913

[16] PRO: HO45/10533-151107/86, 94 and 95

[17] Annual report for Brentry for 1911

[18] Brentry Quarterly report 24 Jan 1916 page 7

[19] printed minutes 24 January 1916, including financial statements

[20] recorded in printed minutes for 22 January 1917

[21] 4th Report of Board of Control, for 1917. *BPP:*1918 xi 569

[22] 1918 XI 569 page 68

[23] see Superintendent's report at Annual Meeting 1 May 1918

[24] Report of the Committee of Management under the MDA, dated October 1917 - Printed minutes of Board of Management 24 October 1917, page 7

[25] Report of Mental Deficiency Committee July 1918 - in printed minutes Board of Management, 22 July 1918, page 6

[26] See Board of Control Annual Report for 1919 *BPP:* 1920 xxi 229

[27] *PRO*: ED50/113 Minute 14/1812 dated 26 March 1914

[28] Wellcome index of Institutions - it closed as a reformatory in 1915.

[29] PRO: HO45/10992/ file 125936/53

[30] PRO: HO45/10992/ file 125936/54

[31] see resolutions 41 of 28 January 1920 and 22 of 21 July 1920

[32] though the annual registers of the NIPRCC give a date of discharge of 1 Nov 1921, all other official reports state 31st Oct

[33] List of Staff and remunerations as at July 1917 - printed minutes Board of Management 23 July 1917, page 13-14

[34] see annual reports of the time

[35] See printed minutes of Board of Management - 1 March 1917, resolution 48

[36] printed minutes Board of Management, 22 July 1918, page 7 and resolution 19 - appointing the committee which comprised the 4 senior officials - Jackson, Field, Burden and Mr Abbott

[37] letter dated 22 Feb 1919. *GLRO:*CJ1/C2

[38] letter dated 28 Feb 1919 from Mather Jackson *GLRO:*CJ1/C2

[39] Letter from Mather Jackson to Gardom dated 28 Feb 1919; *GLRO:* CJ1/C2

[40] described in the Brentry Annual Report for 1919

[41] see report of emergency committee, contained in Brentry Annual report for year ended March 1920

[42] ratified at Annual meeting April 1920 – printed minutes.

[43] recommendation 2 of emergency committee in printed minutes for 23 July 1919

[44] Charity Commission Scheme - Sealed 3 Jan 1922: 4/22 Gloucester, Westbury on Trym, Brentry Certified Inebriate Reformatory - B/78,151.

[45] see Printed minutes of Special Meeting 30 April 1919, pages 11-12.

[46] *PRO*: HO45/10992/file 125936 /41 letter dated 27 Mar 1915

[47] *PRO*: HO45/10992/file 125936 /41 24 Mar 1915

[48] printed minutes 22 July 1918, page 5

[49] Minutes of 30 April 1919, page 12

[50] *GLRO:* CJ1/C2

[51] Ibid

[52] *GLRO:* CJ1/C2 report from the Deputy mayor and Alderman White on their visit to Brentry certified

Institution on 21st June 1922.

[53] *GLRO:* CJ1/C2 memo dated 13 June 1923 with report of Henbury Parish Council from *Daily Press.*

[54] *GLRO:* CJ1/C2 copy leter dated 2 May 1923,

[55] the meeting is detailed in printed minutes for 24 July 1922, pages 4 - 22.

[56] Annual report for Brentry year ended March 1923

[57] The conversion cost £1150. Rather oddly the Annual Report records a debt of gratitude for the building of the workshops to Dr Branthwaite.

[58] Cost £1800 excluding fittings

[59] Inspectors report 16 June 1924, in Brentry Annual report for year ended March 1925

[60] printed minutes 24 July 1922, page 9.

[61] Inspectors report 16 June 1924, in Brentry Annual report for year ended March 1925

[62] See *BRO:* 40686/B/C/1: the building was two storeys, 240 feet by 40 feet, built of concrete, plaster and bricks, lined inside with felt and varnished wood. It was also used as an Officers' mess. The fire was due to a defective flue.

[63] see Brentry Annual report for year ended March 1928, which also has a photograph of it. The opening was covered in the local newspapers.

[64] described on page 5 of Annual Report for Brentry for year ended March 1926

[65] see list of take over and beds on page 17 of 1947 annual report and see bed list in 1930 annual report.

[66] *GLRO:* CJ1/C2

Consolidation

In 1930 Brentry, at 333 inpatients, was still close to the maximum size recommended in 1919. It was rather custodial in nature and was a cheap place to operate. The capital expenditure (£300 per bed) and running costs (£52 per year per patient) were low compared to the costs of other colonies and less than a tenth of equivalent modern costs. The 1930s marked its development into something that is more recognisable as a therapeutic colony.

However this development occurred when there was national pressure to reduce costs and encourage overcrowding. In the 1920s Mental Deficiency colonies were still rather ignored by the government. The government's first main action of the period is said to have occurred when it realised that the cost of opening a bed in a Mental Deficiency colony was higher than working-class housing.[1] It set up the Hedley Committee to look at the costs of operating the colonies and in 1931 this committee made many recommendations to reduce costs[2] ignoring the effect the changes would have on the ideal up-to-date institutions so recently eulogised by another Committee (see Appendix 4). It recommended that Colony sizes be increased to 1000 or more with the beds changed from two to three rows in a dormitory, the wards changed to being semidetached and put closer together to save money on roads and utilities. The overcrowding this induced was not improved until the colonies next hit the news with the scandals of the 1970s.

The two years of 1929 and 1930 saw the loss of two people who were very important in the early life of Brentry. The later was the death of the Rev. Burden. He died at the age of 70, on the 15 May 1930 at Clevedon Hall, from his longstanding Myocarditis.[3] His passing was noted by several obituaries in the national press, and one in the annual report of the Board of Control, but none appeared in the annual report for Brentry. Brentry was thus released from its emotional and managerial ties with the *Inc.NIPRCC* as Harold's successors had little involvement with Brentry except that one of the Committee members of Brentry, C.G. Field Esq. became a trustee of the *NIPRCC.*

The other more silent loss was the retirement of Dr Ormerod in 1929. Though he had worked at Brentry since its foundation his departure is given no special attention in the annual reports. His departure though, did trigger a major change. The Board of Control 'recommended' that to reflect the modern approach to mental deficiency a medical superintendent should replace him rather than a separate superintendent and medical officer. The Board of Control had the power to require that the superintendent be a medical officer so this recommendation was probably interpreted as an order and accepted by the Brentry management committee as it was by many colony committees around the country. To his regret, Mr Lambert's employment was terminated[4] though he departed with a pension. In Lambert's parting report he records the building of the new laundry across the road from the stable wing[5] and his creation of a library of 500 books for the colony by acquiring discarded books from a library. The annual sports day was held on August Bank Holiday 'as is the custom'. In the same year the name of Brentry was changed from *Brentry Certified Institution* to *Brentry Colony*.

Three doctors were interviewed for the new job and Dr R Fitzroy Jarrett (F.R.F.P.S.) was appointed from 1 July 1929, starting at £650 per annum, with accommodation in the main block (on the top floor of the main staircase).[6] Dr Jarrett's employment marked the start of many 'improvements' at Brentry which reflected its change from being a reformatory which contained inmates to being a 'therapeutic' medical institution which treated patients. He initiated changes aimed to prevent 'the impression of punitive detention' and to create a more beneficial environment with the realisation of 'our real aim and object in life as a community of doctors, nurses and patients'.[7] Acting on the advice of Dr Jarrett four staff of the Royal Infirmary were retained as consultants to the colony: a Physician, Surgeon, Ophthalmologist and E.N.T. Surgeon. A dentist was employed as well 'to be of profound benefit to many of our patients whose mouths are in a somewhat deplorable condition'.[8] The evidence of this deplorable state

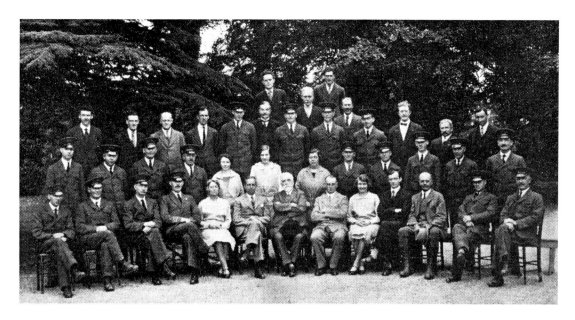

Figure 6.1: The Chairman (Mather Jackson), Hon. Secretary and Staff in 1930

is evident in the photographs of so many edentulous residents over the next 30 years. A fully trained and experienced male nurse was appointed to the 'head post' to aid the adaptation of the junior nursing staff to the new approach and during 1930 the Colony was recognised as a Training School for the Certificate of the Royal Medico-Psychological Association. Dr Jarrett planned the local lecture course and eight of eleven staff passed the exams in May 1931. Soon after this Dr Jarrett was asked to join the Association's education committee, which was an honour achieved by few doctors who worked in Mental Deficiency Colonies. He also revised the medical notes and started the habit of keeping 'full and continuous case notes' with the patients all being re-examined at length.

As with Dr. Fleck, the arrival of a medical superintendent quickly resulted in the colony patients being 'reclassified' along with the blocks: the 'lowest grade' were moved from 'C' block to the lower village, and the most able replaced them as 'better able to appreciate their surroundings'.[9] The Board of Control Inspector who visited at the time, Miss R Darwin, was generally satisfied but recommended commencing a scouting group and developing hostel accommodation.[10] She pointed out that setting aside one of the cottages for the scout group and attaching special privileges to it had occurred at the Manor, Epson and the Royal Eastern Counties' Institution very successfully. Miss Darwin also suggested that Dr Jarrett look at using the patients to build the new workshops and recreation hall as occurred at 'Calderstones and elsewhere'.

January 1931[11] marked the opening of the new Concert Hall 'and cinema' without its orchestral pit (Figure 6.2). The hall was built on the site of the corrugated Iron workshop erected in 1900 and 'recently occupied by Charge Attendant Browne'.[12] New workshops were also built on part of the Kitchen Garden (alongside the stable workshops so that they could share the same toilet facilities). Both were built using patient labour at a cost of almost £4300. The workshops provided two new tailors workrooms and a sewing room (but not the brush-making shop suggested by Dr Jarrett) (Figure 6.3). At the same time the old central dining hall system for the patients was abandoned as their accommodation was altered into 'self contained units'. Prior to this, for the last 30 years the residents had eaten either in a dining room in the old stable block, or else in the lower village in the dining room block built in 1906. The top village's old receiving house had the 11 who normally slept there cleared out to use as an Isolation Hospital for an outbreak of Scarlet fever. It was then adapted to receive up to ten refractory patients[13] with the very high staff ratio of two (plus alarm bell) recommended by the Board of Control inspector.

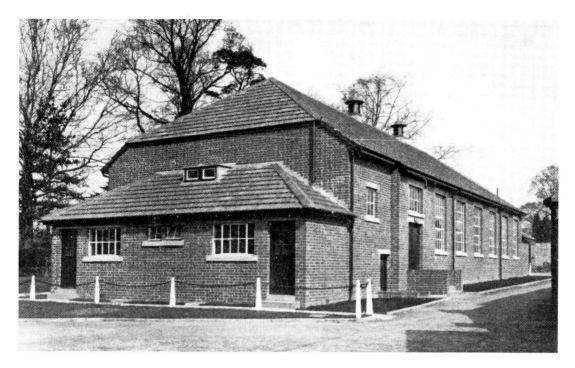

Figure 6.2 The new Concert Hall.

At the same time sport was developed. The teams were given proper colours to wear, instead of the previous night-shirts, and this was noted to improve the keenness of the patients to play and two teams were fielded. One of the first away matches for the football team was with the Bristol City Police. For the next decade the teams all did well, usually winning the majority of their away matches.

The changes effected by Dr Jarrett in his two years as Medical Superintendent were being noticed nationally. The Chairman of the Board of Control visited unofficially in February 1931 'to see progress in the colony'. Soon afterwards Dr Jarrett resigned from Brentry to take up the post of Medical Superintendent at a new large colony being founded by the Kent County Council. However there were 23 applicants for his post at Brentry when it was advertised and as a result a highly regarded man, Dr Gerald Richmond Anderden de Montjoie Rudolf, M.R.C.P, M.R.C.S., D.P.M., D.P.H. was appointed in his stead.[14]

At this time the Royal Medico-Psychological Association published its first substantial book of instruction for Mental Deficiency Nurses: *Manual for Mental Deficiency Nurses.*[15] 'The Green Book' as it came to be known, covers a wide range of topics, but 60% of it is concerned with physical nursing care and anatomy. It sets out the main purposes of the Colony as follows:

1. A training school for mentally defective children or adults for whom suitable training outside is not available.
2. A shelter for those who are homeless, neglected, or otherwise in need of a home and protection.
3. A hospital for those who are of low grade or physically helpless or epileptic, and require nursing care which cannot be provided in their own homes.
4. A place of control for those who are mischievous, destructive, harmful, who are a danger to themselves or to others if left in the community....

With the lower grade the aim must be to render them less dependent members of society by training them in cleanly and independent habits and in the simplest form of manual work; with the medium grade the training may fit them to act as labourers in the unskilled branches of different trades, or to perform simple manual tasks; those of a still higher grade may attain to skilled industrial work.

The valuable qualities of a nurse are listed as: discretion; endurance and cheerfulness; firmness; self-control; honesty of purpose and altruism. His general duties are: cleanliness;

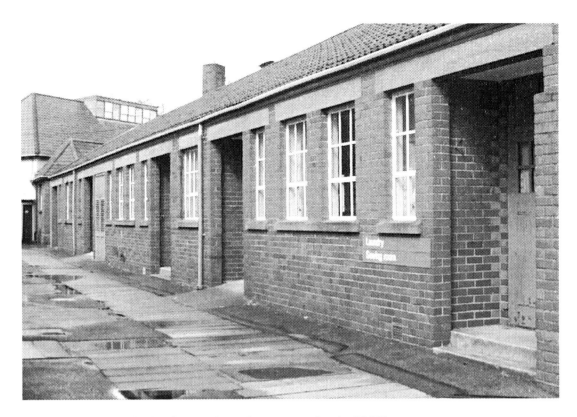

Figure 6.3 The 1931 tailor and sewing rooms (as in 2000).

order and punctuality; discipline and observation. It was clearly thought that a hygienic well-ordered colony was needed to produce physically fit and socially desirable residents.

Dr Gerald Richmond Anderden de Montjoie Rudolf

Dr Rudolf was paid on similar terms to Dr Jarrett.[16] He had previously been an assistant medical officer in London at the Cane Hill and Claybury Mental Hospitals. In 1934 he was awarded 'a special prize for research in mental disease' by the Royal Medico-Psychological Association, following his co-authorship of the report *The relative mortality of Cancer in the general population and in the mental hospitals of England and Wales.*[17] He and Dr Jarrett were two of the few mental deficiency superintendents who were appointed to any committee in the R.M.P.A. An old member of staff remembers him as being a shortish, very polite man who was also firm. 'His first aim was always patients. Patients, patients and patients - he was very good.'

Dr Rudolf's first year started with vetting the library books. Half were judged to be unsuitable. The Head Nurse formed a social club and some of the patients started to keep pets. To encourage good behaviour, two blocks in each village were set apart for the use of the better behaved, in which they received special privileges. In addition the iron bars were removed from the old windows in the lower village.[18] The old stable workshops were also converted during 1932, and opened in March 1933 as the ground floor ward Shackleton for well behaved patients and the upper floor used for female nurse accommodation (after appointing a sister and female staff nurse).[19]

Dr Jarrett had complained that the 'new' hospital on the top two floors of the three-storey annex was unsuitable for what it was being used for. It was not just used as a hospital. No nursing staff lived or slept on the wards at Brentry, unlike most Lunatic Asylums where staff lived in rooms on the wards. In Brentry a night nurse toured the wards, making it easy to abscond and difficult to care for people who were incontinent at night. The Hospital was the only ward staffed at night so it was used for both the physically ill and some of the absconders. All cases needing a diagnosis of their 'insanity' were placed there as well. Under Dr Rudolf the old receiving house in the upper village was converted from being a unit for refractory patients into a hospital, with an extension to isolate tubercular cases. With the opening of the new hospital the old hospital was converted during 1933 to a new block 'Darwin'. The result was an increase in the beds in the Colony to 367 by March 1934.

Dr Rudolf continued his policy of classifying and rewarding good behaviour. He moved the people with epilepsy into the upper village and moved 'lower grades' to the lower. The lower village had a block for patients with good behaviour for 6 months. Each village then had a block for 12 months good behaviour. Top grade patients progressed from here to the two blocks of the Main Building, Darwin and Shackleton (known by patients as 'The Grades' for a long time afterwards). Here each ward was run by a committee of three patients who were responsible for the ward's cleanliness, discipline and for reporting misbehaviour. Each committee met weekly and sent minutes to Dr Rudolf. A nurse visited once daily to issue stores and others visited at irregular times. The patients of these blocks had free parole on the estate, whereas others did not.[20] Misdemeanours were enquired into closely by Dr de M. Rudolf and his nurses:

> Frequently, witnesses are brought forward by each of the parties. These witnesses may have been bribed by cigarettes. Enquiries are often carried over several days and may include the interview of perhaps a dozen persons. So much depends, from the patient's point of view, upon the result of the enquiry [as the miscreant will be moved to a lower grade ward] that no stone must be left unturned in order to reach a just conclusion.[21]

During 1932 two thirds of the patients of the entire Colony were sent out of the grounds on parole with no complaints from the public. Similarly earlier there was an outing for 258 patients to the matinee at Bristol Hippodrome where 'the members of the public in other parts of the house were unaware of the patients'. Over the next year the parole system was refined with the best patients aspiring to live in the Grades with individual parole on the estate and parole off the estate in parties of three.

In 1932 the Board of Control commented yet again on the low staffing levels - for example in 'B' block in lower village one nurse had to look after 24 low grade patients, many of whom required his attention when toileting. They also pointed out the relatively high number of injuries happening (80 assaults in 6 months) as evidence of inadequate supervision. After this report the Committee agreed to the employment of an extra five staff and a steward. The first female nurses were appointed at this time and all the new staff received additional training before appointment. This training was usually how to play a musical instrument as much as how to look after the patients.

A scout group was formed during the end of 1932[22] as recommended by Miss Darwin from the Board of Control. This was not seen as radical for the scout movement had been in mental deficiency institutions for 8 years by then. By March 1934[23] 51 patients had passed the Tenderfoot Test for Scouts and a drum and bugle band had been formed for the Scout Group.

Dr Rudolf further refined his method of behaviour grouping with gradation of work passes and parole dependent on behaviour.[24] The Colony also decided to permit the admission of Roman Catholic Patients in the same year that the Bishop of Malmesbury visited to confirm 15 candidates in the colony chapel. In 1934 the gates of the 'tradesmen's entrance', the main practical entrance to the colony by the reception bungalow, were replaced with some iron gates donated from a 'Mansion House' of Lord Raglan and called the 'Raglan Gates'.

On 4 July 1934 the Management Board redeemed its two outstanding mortgages[25] including that of the NIPRCC, and took out a fresh loan of £15000 at 4% from the Royal Liver Friendly Society.[26] To do this they paid for a valuation of the site which was £46,500 if reused as an institution and £27,000 as building land.[27] More money[28] was borrowed to install a central heating system throughout the colony, to improve life on the blocks. At this time a new boiler house was built next to the old engine house in the old kitchen garden. This building has the date 1936 above its doors.

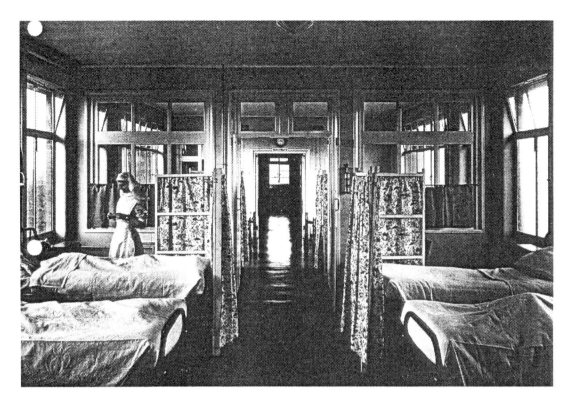

Figure 6.4: Mather Jackson Hospital: Owen ward from Abbots ward.

At the end of 1935 a new Hospital was opened joined to the old one (formerly the women's receiving house). Called the Mather Jackson Hospital after the long-serving chairman, it had two wards, Abbots and Owen (Figure 6.4) named after two trustees, one for high and one for low grades.[29] In addition it contained a dental and outpatient department and dispensary. The Isolation and tubercular wards[30] were in the old receiving house attached to it, and platforms were constructed for the tubercular patient's beds to be wheeled into the sunshine. The tubercular cases used the veranda by day and slept in the day accommodation.[31] In addition a mortuary was constructed attached to the end of the conjoined blocks in the upper village. A staff mess was built in the lower village, containing a Charge Nurse's Room, general mess room, kitchen, cloakroom and lavatories.

When the Board of Control Inspector visited in January 1936, the Colony was in a form virtually unchanged until 1970 (see figure 6.5). The new engineer's workshops and boiler house were being built by the old engine room. There were 371 patients in the colony on 31 March 1936 including one private patient - 'an elderly man who now appears to have no relations in this country' who had been there for many years. In the Main Building, Darwin contained 34 'boys', and was larger than Shackleton. In the Upper Village the conjoined block 'B' was a vast warehouse that contained 118 of the less well behaved, including 34 'epileptics', whilst the adjacent 'new' 'C' block on the site of Warwick, had 62 patients. The new hospital contained a total of 26 beds. In addition there was the original Infirmary of 1899, now extended as block 'A'. In the Lower village there were 5 blocks: 'A' for boys with 6 months good behaviour (23); 'B' for lowest grades admitted (26); 'C' slept 14 and also provided the day space for 'D' which was used only for sleeping. 'E' block held 24. The entire colony, comprising 8 staffed and 2 un-staffed wards was supervised by about 28 male day nurses and 7 male night nurses, with 2 female day nurses and one night female nurse working in the infirmary. Many of the day staff ran the workshops and about half or less of the staff were left to cover the hospital in the evenings and at weekends, which limited the opportunity for recreation. Despite this there were active football and cricket teams who played most weeks of the season, as well as the scouts and one or two patients played in a staff orchestra. There was only one annual sports day and one annual colony

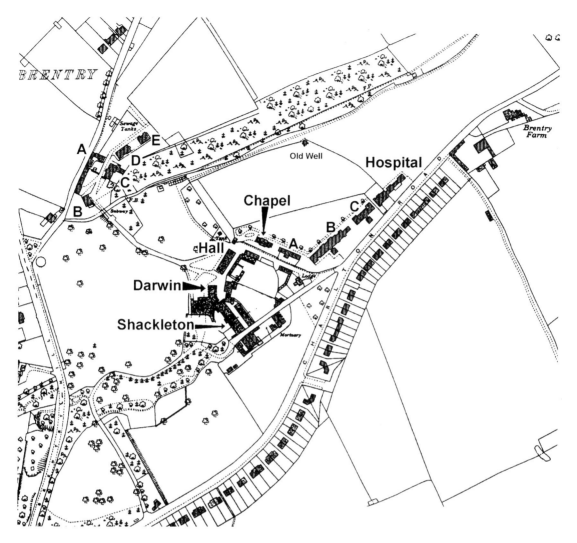

Figure 6.5: Brentry in 1935, with block names – note that workshops opposite Chapel have not been built.

outing, whose venues included the Zoo, Cheddar Gorge, Sand Bay and 'visiting a local pageant'. by 1939 the colony was using a more permanent holiday camp at Aust. There seems to have been two or three patients absconding every year. Each year about 40 patients were sent on 'Holiday Leave' (leave of up to 3 months), and about 40 patients sent out to live and work on licence (leave longer than 3 months), prior to discharge. The behaviour of patient was still being rewarded by where they lived in the colony and the degree of parole they were allowed. The Colony does seem to have accommodated a more able group than in the 1980s as only 20 or so are noted to be incontinent at night. The feeling gained is that many of the patients were minor delinquents, sent a distance from home by their funding authorities. On arrival the patents were escorted everywhere and only after 3 months of good reports were they allowed to go from the block to work and back unescorted on the issue of a 'work pass'. At six months they moved to a better ward and allowed to leave the grounds in groups of three but were not allowed parole around the colony alone until there had been 9 months good behaviour. They returned to the Blocks to eat their meals. The Colony continued to be surrounded by high walls and manned gates and all the patients were detained under the Mental Deficiency Act.

As with all colonies and lunatic asylums, the colony tried to be as self sufficient as possible. The employment activities remained relatively unchanged over many years. Some reports that that most of the patients were found employment around the colony with only 5 or 10% felt not to be employable, though many must have performed very simple domestic tasks and the numbers employed seems to have depended on whether simple domestic duties were seen as employment. Employment was stated to have included

> 'care of horses, cows, pigs and poultry, boot and shoe making and repairing, fancy leather work and wool rug making [initiated by Mrs Jarrett], basket work, raffia work, chair and stool making, coir mat making, laundry work, tailoring, sewing, darning, shirt-making, stocking making, wood chopping, stoking, carpentering, stone-work and brick-laying, road-making [and later tarmac laying], house decorating, domestic work, clerical work and typing.[32]

There also was gardening, helping in the fields and kitchens, net-making and fretwork. A few years later 198 patients were performing formal work:

> 33 whose trade training is sufficient to enable them to work with the tradesmen on the maintenance staff; 43 receive instruction in basket making, raffia weaving and rug-making - 12 are capable of high quality work unaided; 57 work on the farm and garden - 30 as key-men, 27 as labourers; 20 work in the laundry, 18 with the seamstress and 16 work with the tailor; 11 work in the shoe-maker's shop, making all the footwear used in the Institution.[33]

During the 1930s the cost of the food and provisions for Brentry was cut, from £4s 7d per inmate per week in 1929 to 3s 10d in 1939. The annual reports make no specific mention of this or of any change in the diets used at the Colony and it can only be assumed that this cost reduction was due to the economies of the increased population of the colony and improved use of the land. However this was a time when there was central governmental pressure to reduce expenditure and there may well have been deliberate bearing down on the costs of the Colony.

The year 1936 marked the start of recruitment problems. Dr Rudolf resigned on the 31 July 1936, though he remained a visiting doctor to the Colony for many years afterwards. Until at least 1957 he wrote an annual research and publications report for the annual report as 'Visiting Consultant Psychiatrist'.

The Board had trouble recruiting a successor, having to increase the salary to £800 pa. to recruit Dr James Johnston Mason M.B., Ch.B. from the navy. He is said to have been a very firm man who liked a military approach such as short haircuts. The residents would quickly get out of the way if they saw him coming. The Head Nurse Mr W T Williams also resigned, to take up the post of Superintendent in a Yorkshire Institution for Defectives. He was succeeded by Mr E C Urch from Hortham Colony.[34] The growth of local industry meant that several nursing staff left and there were difficulties replacing them, due to the long hours and low pay.

The arrival of Dr Mason led to the renaming of the blocks during 1937 to eliminate 'the drab system of lettered "blocks".'[35] The new 'villas' were now named after inspirational men:

In the lower village: A: Kipling; B: Baden-Powell; C: Haig; D: Allenby; E: Shakespeare

In the Upper Village: A: Dickens; B: Jellicoe; C: Wellington.

Baden Powell Villa was so named as it housed a reformed boy scout troop.

> The Boy Scout movement was revised early last year with a view to creating a really effective troop. The movement is beyond the concepts of low grade defectives, and though now the troop numbers only 37, it is more comparable with an average school-boy troop in regard to scouting "lore". The troop formed the nucleus of the summer holiday camp, laying out the site, pitching, assisting in patrolling, and finally striking. A large permanent Scout camp is being prepared at Shirehampton by the District Boy Scout Association and our troop was invited to share in this work. Several enjoyable Sunday afternoon trips have been made to this site by parties from out troop and we believe their services have been appreciated.

Most of the Scouts are quartered in Baden-Powell Villa, from which they are distributed during working hours. It is expected that their standard of behaviour should act as an example to those others with whom they mingle while at work and recreation.'[36]

The inspector reported in 1938 that

Formerly nearly everyone was a scout but now the name applies only to those able to appreciate the advantages of the movement. 24 scouts in Baden Powell, 13 'tenderfoots' in upper village [presumably in the 'Grades'].[37]

The War

The war brought many changes and pressures which are best introduced by the report of Dr Mason:

Most of the Staff and many patients felt the growing anxiety of the general community becoming more personal in its application as time passed. Early in summer [1939] the need for air-raid shelters was the talk of everyone. Work was accordingly begun. Anti-gas respirators soon were being issued and A.R.P. classes organised. A few regular Army reservists on the Staff were quietly departing to rejoin the Colours. Later on thirteen [over a third] of the nursing and instructional staff departed overnight as members of the Army Supplementary Reserve. Next day came the War. Work on our air-raid precautions became our sole endeavour, the patients responding with vigour and enthusiasm to the need for work, work and more work. Ten wholly underground shelters were excavated, [in front of Wellington Villa] mostly out of rocky ground, concrete lined and roofed, and ready for emergency occupation within few weeks of the coming of War. The black-out arrangements were at first makeshift and caused internal gloom by day as well as by night. … I must compliment the Staff on the way they carried out evening and night duties under very unpleasant conditions, and give praise to the patients for the way they preserved decorum and order *and* their good spirits during those first gloomy months. As time has passed conditions have become more normal, so that now our present troubles are confined to the continuous depletion of the Staff, particularly trained young male nurses and the difficulty of obtaining suitable elderly men to replace them. The gradual rise in the number of patients in the Colony, due in part to war restrictions on accommodation in other Institutions, is placing a [additional] growing strain on the depleted … Staff.[38]

The changes affected all parts of life at the Colony. Twenty six of the staff had left, including the Head and Deputy Head Male Nurses. The man appointed to be Head Male Nurse was Mr L Browne who had worked at the Colonies as an instructor for years, occupying the Iron Hut prior to the Concert Hall being built. The two who replaced the deputy were both beyond military age. Ten probationers were appointed and fortunately 11 of the male nurses passed the R.M.P.A. final examinations as mental deficiency nurses. However, the problem continued with the continual loss of staff and in 1943 the medical superintendent reported problems due to 'recruiting attendants who are seldom physically capable, and not always mentally so'. The loss of the nurse tutor meant that the nursing school had to be temporarily closed during 1943.[39]

The accommodation had to be enlarged to accommodate the increase in patients and so Haig was altered to take another 11 residents. In addition a larger than usual quantity of redecoration and minor alterations was needed and was performed by the residents and staff.

Due to the changes and demands of work the weight of the (more able) upper village residents fell by 8 pounds to 9 stone 1 pound in the first 6 months of the war. Dr Mason though, noted that the Epileptic patients seemed to be better for the increase in outdoor activities and were having much fewer fits. The evening meals were rearranged to combine tea and supper into a meal at 5.45pm combined with 'early bedding'. The food used started to include many more dishes that only needed heating in the Colony kitchens. A patient's canteen and shop that started prior to the war continued despite the other changes.

Most of the patients were well behaved despite the lack of staff, no doubt helped by the increase in exhausting physical activity. In the early months three patients were secluded but in addition, due to the staffing problems the Hospital Block was used for a multitude of cases that needed higher supervision, including new patients and patients returning from absconding, as well as medically ill people. It started to resemble the old Darwin hospital. The next year, due to nurse anxiety about its vulnerability, the Hospital block was moved in the next year to the main building (apart from the TB cases) using an old store room and chemical toilets. In addition another room in the Main building was changed to a casualty room for any injuries in the colony or locally.[40]

Parole outside of the Colony was completely suspended for the first two months of the war, probably due to staff shortages. However in March 1940 there were still 50 patients out on licence. More of the patients worked around the Colony and Dr Mason lists 382 in occupations, with 14 'low-grades' chopping and bundling firewood (though this stopped in 1940 due to the supply of old railway sleepers running out[41]) and 26 in 'kindergarten occupations'.

As the war progressed patients started to obtain work outside the colony. In 1942 Dr Mason reported that 13 patient were now in private employment and the following year another 18 were at the new agricultural hostels where they lived with a warden but provided labour for the neighbouring farms. This grew over the war years until by the 1945 report, there were 36 on licence working in the agricultural hostels and another 30 working in Bristol in paid work.

Recreational activities were maintained though initially matches with other teams stopped as most external teams had been disbanded and the colony had to find other teams to play against.

With the war though, the Scout troop came into its own. The loss of staff continued so that 30 staff left during 1940 leaving 14 male staff for the whole colony in November 1940. The Scouts started to help the staff by providing patrols and supervising the gates at the weekend. Unfortunately they themselves were disbanded in 1943 due to lack of staff to manage and instruct them.[42]

Twenty six episodes of absconding occurred in the first year of the war, in part boosted by several repeat absconders. Absconding continued to be an issue throughout the war, with a group of about 8 residents repeatedly absconding. Dr Mason suggested that this was in part due to the distance many patients were from their families combined by the open nature of the Colony and worsened by the lack of staff. The patients generally coped well with the lack of discipline, as in 1943 Dr Mason pointed out that 'control of a disciplinary nature is virtually absent at present since the skeleton staff cannot be spread over all interests, but as a whole the conduct of patients has been good.'

The end of the war brought an employment boom in Bristol. Patients started to abscond again to take advantage of this booming open employment market. Seventy seven absconded in 1946. However patients still based in Brentry found that many places of work were now closed to Brentry patients to cater for men returning from the war. The agricultural hostels in Gloucestershire, which had provided work for many patients during the war, closed over the next 10 years. By 1948 only 22 patients were in outside work.

The end of the war brought back many staff and staff numbers rose to 42. However the employment boom made mental deficiency nursing a very unattractive proposition. Several of the qualified staff left to work elsewhere. The colony had to pay most of its untrained staff at the higher, experienced rate to compete with local industry. They justified this by saying that military service formed appropriate experience.

The end of the war also brought demands and plans for new wards and workshops, a staff recreation room and new buildings to separate the superintendent's accommodation from the administration offices. It was agreed to raise a mortgage to fund these but the post-war economies scuppered the plans. As Dr Mason wrote: 'our turn is a long way off'.[43]

The 1947 annual report commemorated the end of the Management Board of Brentry by a short history of the institution, detailing the contributions made by various councils and omitting all mention of the RVH, Rev. Burden or the *NIPRCC* except to state that

> Largely at the instance of the late Rev. Harold Nelson Burden and the Officers of the Gloucestershire County Council, it was decided to acquire the lands upon which the Colony now stands.[44]

Notes

[1] See Mathew Thomson: *The Problem of Mental Deficiency.* Oxford: Clarendon Press, 1998. Pages 130ff

[2] *Report of the Departmental Committee on Colonies for Mental Defective (Hedley Report).* London: HMSO, 1931 [not a Command paper]

[3] Death certificate. (in Burden Trust deposition at *B.R.O.*) this certificate gives age as 71.

[4] see end of his report, page 20 of Brentry Annual report for year ended March 1929

[5] with tenders for building and equipment totalling £2667

[6] three doctors were Dr Ferguson, Dr Jarrett and Dr Wyatt; appointment and condition on page 5 of Annual Report year ended March 1929

[7] Brentry Annual report for year ended March 1930, page 20

[8] Ann Report Mar 1930, page 23 - Med. Supt.'s report

[9] Board of Control inspectors report in Annual report ending March 1930

[10] *Ibid.* report of R Darwin visit of 27 February 1930

[11] Concert Hall illustrated in Ann Report ending March 1931

[12] Annual report of general committee, page 7 of Annual report for 1930 for Brentry.

[13] Board of Control's report Ann Report ended Mar 1931. Block capable of receiving 10, 5 in single rooms, and would need 2 staff and an alarm bell -suggesting isolated. *Also notes that only one female employed - a seamstress*

[14] the other candidate interviewed was Dr Rodger. The shortlist was interviewed by the management board at their Annual General Meeting - Ann Report ended March 1931

[15] RMPA: *Manual for Mental Deficiency Nurses.* London: Bailliere & Co, 1931.

[16] £650 per annum with an extra £150 for rations he could not obtain from the colony and £30 for laundry if the colony could not do it. He was not allowed to have a private practice.

[17] report published in *Journal of Mental Science* April 1934.

[18] foregoing from Annual Report ended March 1932

[19] The conversion cost about £1100 as part of the walls and roof needed rebuilding.

[20] see Brentry Colony: *Medical and Administrative Reports 1933.* (Bristol, Henry Hill Ltd: 1933) 'Behaviour Grouping', page 12

[21] Medical superintendents report in 1933 Annual report

[22] Ann Report end March 1933 - Inspectors report

[23] Annual report 1934

[24] see Medical report (page 20) in Annual report for year ending March 1934

[25] £4820 at 6% (from the original purchase) and £6400 at 4% (from NIPRCC)

[26] deeds of loans at Bevan Ashfords. Event discussed in Annual report ending March 1934

[27] Amongst deeds at Bevan Ashford.

[28] 14 Feb 1936 further loan of £11,800 from Royal Liver Friendly Society at 4% repayable over 15 years.

[29] photo in Annual Report ended March 1936

[30] the veranda is illustrated in G de M. Rudolf & A E Oaten: 'A note upon the roofs of Closed verandas' *Nosokomeion* (1933) IV/4:663

[31] in Inspectors 1941 report (see Annual Report)

[32] Medical superintendent's report for 1932.

[33] Report of Inspector of Board of Control, in Brentry Annual Report for 1938.

[34] Ann Report ending March 1936. The watertower that existed by the concert hall, may have been built in 1936 as a drawing of it dated 1936 exists in the plans department. This may reflect a desire to improve the water pressure or fire fighting capabilities. At the same time the engineering and maintenance shops were built, as they have the date 1936 on them.

[35] Ann report ending March 1938 page 18

[36] Ann Report year ending March 1938 page 18

[37] Ann report ending March 38

[38] Medical Superintendent's report in annual report for 1940.

[39] Medical Supt's report for year ended March 1944

[40] Board of Control visit Nov 1940 in 1941 Annual report

[41] Board of Control visit Nov 1940 in 1941 Annual report

[42] Medical Supt's report for year ended March 1944

[43] 1948 annual report

[44] Annual report for 1947, page 15

The Start of the National Health Service

When the National Health Service was first planned the Mental Illness Hospitals and Mental Deficiency Colonies were not included within the new service.[1] The Board of Control who supervised them argued that this would not be possible until the Mental Health legislation was reformed. However most bodies supported the idea of closer working between Mental Health and other Health Services and at the last minute, with the agreement of the Board of Control, the Mental Health Services and Mental Deficiency services were included in the 1944 White Paper on the new NHS. This paper proposed that all the hospitals and health services should be administered under local authority joint boards. In the case of mental deficiency the prospect was that at long last the administration of all the various bodies providing a service, including the public assistance committee, county mental deficiency committee and county education committee would be brought under one administrative structure. However the Bill was revised and the National Health Service Act that was passed set up Regional Hospital Boards [RHB's] separate to local authorities. Other radical welfare legislation set up the precursor of the modern welfare state by abolishing the remains of the old Poor Law and substituting a new system of welfare operated by the local authorities, who would also run community services for people with mental deficiency. The National Health Act allowed the NHS authorities to run some of these community services linked to the new mental deficiency 'hospitals'. However the Regional Hospital Boards, as the name implied, tended to focus on hospitals and not community services, particularly when financial pressures meant that any money not tied to bricks and mortar was under threat.[2] The RHB's set up new local hospital boards who took over and administered a motley collection of cottage hospitals, asylums run by local authorities, famous charity hospitals and hostels run by voluntary bodies. By this measure virtually the entire residential accommodation used by 'mental defectives' was brought into the health service and removed from the control of the Local Authorities and Boards of Guardians. The idea of a joint service integrating hospitals, health community services and local authority services had to wait another 50 years, until 2001, before it was again included in government policy.

A good example of the effect of the take-over is the hospital boards for the mental deficiency services around Bristol. To the south in Somerset, Bedminster Workhouse and Yatton Hall stopped being operated by Somerset Mental Deficiency Committee to become part of the Sandhill Park Hospital Management Committee based by Taunton. The Stoke Park Group of Colonies, operated by the Incorporation of the National Institutions for Persons Requiring Care and Control, was so large it was made a hospital group in its own right. Brentry Colony, run by its Consortium of Local Authorities, was merged with Bristol Mental Deficiency Committee's purpose built colony, Hortham, to form the Hortham-Brentry Hospital Group. To it were added an odd group of hostels:

> Chasefield Laundry Home and the Royal Fort Homes, both run by the Bristol Preventative Mission,

> St Mary's Home, Painswick, a private charity established in 1893.

> The Shurdlington and Newent Agricultural Hostels in Gloucesterhire, operated by the National Association for Mental Health.

> The House of Help and the Old Rectory run in Bath by the Bath Preventative Mission,

> Rockhall School, Bath which was run by the Bath Municipal Charity Trustees and derived from an ancient leper hospital and the first modern idiot school in England founded in 1846.[3]

Brentry Colony contrasted strongly with Hortham. Brentry was a colony that had few links with Bristol and sat as an isolated community in Bristol. Its inmates were all men from outside Bristol and many returned to their own areas when they left. Most of the staff lived on site or in houses close to the colony. The Board of Management was nominated by a group of County or Borough Councils and their Annual General Meeting was convened in London. Hortham was a larger colony in Almondsbury that was owned and run by Bristol City Council with many of the staff commuting from Bristol and almost all the inmates being linked with the area.

Brentry started being called Brentry Hospital in September 1949[4] to reflect the fact that it was now a part of a health service. However the attitudes of the authorities did not change as rapidly and the name 'Colony' was still used in some documents until March 1953. The ancillary institutions and hostels were added to the group in 1949. Soon after this, on the 15 January 1950, Brentry was formally demoted by being designated ancillary to Hortham. The Group Headquarters and medical superintendent were now based at Hortham with Dr Mason at Brentry downgraded to being deputy medical superintendent. However the main group management committee did not travel as far out of Bristol as Hortham but met away from both hospitals in the city centre.

Early Staff changes

Life for the nurses at Brentry Colony in 1948 was not very attractive though it was not remarkably worse than life in other colonies. The male staff wore serge uniform suits and peaked caps with the letters BC on the front, almost unchanged from the inebriate colony days of 1900 and not due to change until 1970. They wore white protective sleeves over the arms of the suits when they were performing dirty tasks such as serving food, and wore white coats for more dirty tasks. They were responsible for the suits and had to make them last. They worked long shifts with day shifts lasting from 7.30 in the morning to 8.00pm. They worked 4 days on and 2 days off in strict sequence, with 3 months of the year doing night shifts which lasted from 7.30pm to 8.00am. They worked a 60 hour week and there was no additional pay for night or evening work or for overtime. Pay was generally less than that of local semi-skilled workers in industry, who could expect to work a shorter 48 hour week.

During the daytime there were usually 2 staff on a ward, but there could be three for the larger wards, though in practice this often meant that there were two for much of the time. This meant that there could be 2 staff for 70 patients, many of whom were incontinent and needed washing and dressing. 'Dangerous' activities such as shaving would be performed by staff, with the blades counted out and counted back. Everything was counted – the patients, food, cutlery and tools. When patients went to work, or therapy, the staff generally had to accompany them to boost the number of staff in the therapy sessions. This could lead to little protests, such as the nurse who hated gardening who planted all his bulbs together in one single pit to speed up his task. The 'punishment' for nurses was to be placed on 'Gate Duty' manning the entrance to the Hospital. The gates themselves had gone, given up as part of the war effort.

Staff did not approach the doctors who worked on the site. Nurses were expected to refer matters to the chief male nurse who would discuss any concerns with the medical staff. Most months a member of staff would have their glasses broken in an 'incident' and a straitjacket was used for one or two of the more aggressive patients, for periods of up to 2 hours at a time. Staff could however control the patients by regulating their access to cigarettes or to social events. This could lead to discontent and many assaults on staff went unreported.

Just as the hospital wards were decrepit and in urgent need of replacement so the staff cottages were frequently felt to be in desperate need of repair and upgrade. But as with the wards, the Hospital rarely had the money to do the necessary work. Indeed in 1955 the Committee raided the Hospital Amenities Fund to carry out the urgent work as the RHB had not provided the money.[5]

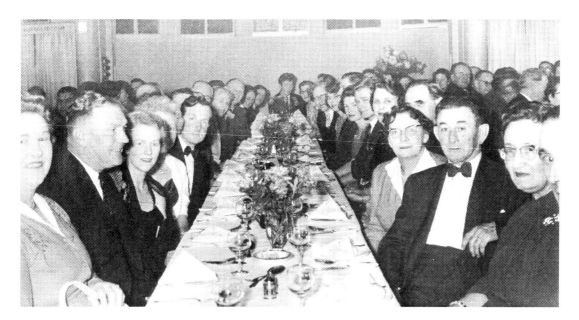

Figure 7.1: Staff Meal 1958

The end result of all this was that the staffing at Brentry was almost always below official strength. At times of high local unemployment recruitment was better but usually the management committee could not be choosy about whom it accepted onto the staff. For much of the time some of the deficiency was filled by staff being allowed to work after their official retirement age but at times in the 1950s this meant that 10% of the staff were over retirement age.

During 1949 three Nursing Assistants left to go to Stoke Park to train as nurses, in order to increase their immediate and long term pay. This made the house committee suggest that they restart the nurse training school at Brentry.[6] Dr Mason as Medical Superintendent of Brentry discussed the matter with the Medical Superintendent of Hortham and they agreed that Brentry could develop a training school attached to Hortham's existing school either with the nurses attending school at Hortham or with a tutor from Hortham visiting Brentry. The General Nursing Council visited Brentry and it was decided to build some pre-fabricated buildings for a school building at Brentry. Brentry Colony was approved as a Nurses Training School in March 1950 and by the end of the year five staff were enrolled as students.[7] Even so, in 1951 it was reported that there were only 20 qualified, 25 unqualified and 5 student nurses looking after over 400 patients and that a further 15 staff were needed to introduce a planned new 'shift' system requested by the staff. As a result the shift system was not revised and the nurses continued to have to work 6 hours overtime a week.[8]

Two years later, with the growth of local industry, the staff shortages worsened, and it was impossible to recruit nursing assistants. As a result less able 'ward orderlies' were employed in their stead.[9] The shortage was made worse by the fact that most student nurses were now leaving before they qualified because their pay and working conditions were worse than those in local industry.[10]

The staff morale was not helped by the downgrade of Brentry to being an ancillary hospital. Dr Mason left soon after his downgrade but he was replaced by the young and energetic Dr Alan Heaton-Ward. He wrote booklet on Mental Deficiency for the nurses of the group, in collaboration with Dr Lyons, the Superintendent at Hortham. This proved a great success so it was published in March 1953 and eventually ran to five editions over the next 31 years. The other status person was Charles Hallas, who as Chief Male Nurse, published a widely read book on 'Nursing the Mentally Subnormal'. Like Dr Heaton-Ward's book this book ran

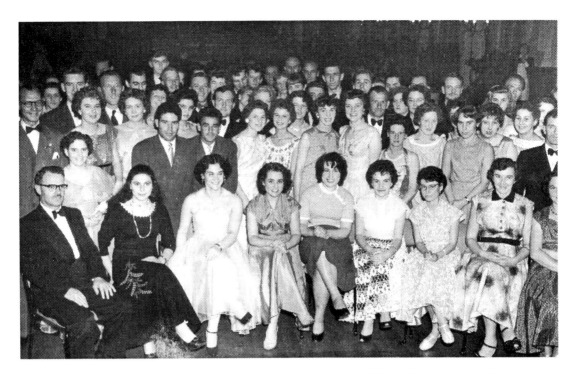

Figure 7.2: Staff Dance about 1958 – Mr Dagger, Chief Male Nurse, is on the left.

to several editions and became a standard text nationally .

One administrative change that occurred during the 1950s was the growth of the power of the new Hospital Group Secretaries, over that of the medical superintendent. This is commented on by Dr. Heaton-Ward, in his reminiscences on Stoke Park, where he describes the conflicts that arose by the end of the decade over who was managed by whom and who controlled clinical staff. At Brentry the growth of power was such that in the 1957 annual report the Group Secretary started giving his own report parallel to that of the Management Committee and of the Medical Superintendent.[11]

During the 1950s there were annual staff dinners and dances, of which some photographs survive (Figures 7.1 and 7.2).

Changes for the Patients

A feature of most publicity about Brentry is how newspaper articles are so complimentary about the colony. Most descriptions reassuringly told people what a wonderful life the residents led. Until the managers publicised the poor conditions in 1969, no newspaper article implies that the colony needs any improvement and must have reassured anyone placing their son in the hospital. One example of this is a newspaper article published for Christmas 1955:[12]

> Resident at the hospital are 436 patients; 21, still certified under the Mental Deficiency Acts, are on licence from the hospital, either to relatives, friends or employers, and 23 more go out daily to work with local employers.
> **It cannot be too strongly stated that none of the patients is dangerous. None is mentally ill.**
> They are people born with slight defects in their mental capacity - people who can be helped by giving them work and responsibility, leisure and pleasure, good food and understanding, recreation and as much freedom as possible.
> And all brought about by a staff with a gift for understanding their problems.

> Rehabilitation is the keynote. A number of patients have been sent to the Industrial Rehabilitation Unit at Fishponds...many are employed in the hospital itself – ... In the shoeshop 20 men work under a shoemaker – instructor, turning out from the raw skins a dozen new pairs a week – and repairing 40 more. Everything is used; there is no waste. Odd pieces are turned into such things as studs for football boots.
>
> In the sewing-room between 400 and 500 pairs of socks are darned every week. And a further 70 are knitted every fortnight. ... in the tailors shop around 600 pieces come in for repair every week.
>
> New suits are made – from beginning to end. Dungarees and overalls for use in the hospital are made up. Again a qualified instructor patiently supervises the work. The laundry takes care of upwards of 6,000 pieces each week.
>
> In the kitchens the dishes for a balanced weekly menu are prepared in huge ovens. A sample menu: Boiled ham, creamed potatoes, beans; apple tart and custard. ...
>
> Brushes, baskets, jig-saws, lamp-shades, dish-cloths – all, and more, are products of the occupational therapy side....
>
> Until recently farming was another hospital pursuit; but now, with the decision of the Ministry of Health to curtail hospital farming and the consequent sale of stock, efforts are concentrated on intensive market gardening....
>
> All [Villas] contain radio and TV sets. ... other forms [of entertainment] include concerts by local players almost every Saturday, and weekly film shows – all held in the concert hall.
>
> Instructional classes in physical training, club swinging, eurythmics and badminton are held, as well as educational classes for high-grade patients.
>
> A football team playing in the Church of England League, a cricket team and sports events complete the activity in the hospital.

However despite this public image of a warm comfortable and productive life, in reality life was as hard for the patients at the start of the NHS as for the nurses. Life had not changed for many years. The wards were large and crowded and there was often not enough seating for all the patients to sit down at once. Clothes were not personalised and the clothing was still institutional hard wearing grey tweed suits that were made in the tailor's shop. One member of staff might have to get up to 40 patients up in the morning so there was hard work, though many patients had their 'Queenies' to help them. Other patients would be given the role of 'lookout' – announcing to the staff whenever someone was approaching the ward. Baths only occurred twice a week, in communal bathrooms that had several baths under the inspection of one member of staff. There were five baths in one room on Haig, but those of Shackleton were single though they had to be used by the patients of Darwin once a week as there was no bath on Darwin. Washing and shaving occurred in queues, with any razor blade issued to staff expected to last for 6 to 8 patient shaves. Any new patient had to lose any sense of modesty very quickly. The speed of washing and dressing meant that no-one had time to sort out appropriate sizes from the communal clothing supply, so many walked around relying on their belts to hold up trousers.

Meals were now eaten on each villa, rather than communal dining halls, with the food brought down from the central kitchen by van. The food was basic. No one was allowed to start their meal until the room was quiet, which could take 20 minutes. Grace was then said and the patients were then allowed to start the food, however cold it had become. Utensils were counted in and out and no one left the dining area until all was accounted for and the room was again quiet and grace said. Food such as butter was strictly rationed, and one staff recalls being puzzled at the loss of butter, until he discovered that the patient who put the butter out was hiding some behind his chair by sticking it to the yellow walls. The dormitories were crowded and few wards had night staff based on them. Most wards were visited at set times by roaming night staff and nocturnal abuse between patients must have been very prevalent and hard to detect by staff. It was recognised by staff that in the exclusively male setting of the Hospital many of the patients had formed supportive partnerships that could include a sexual relationship. Few of the wards were locked at night, in part a reflection of the lack of

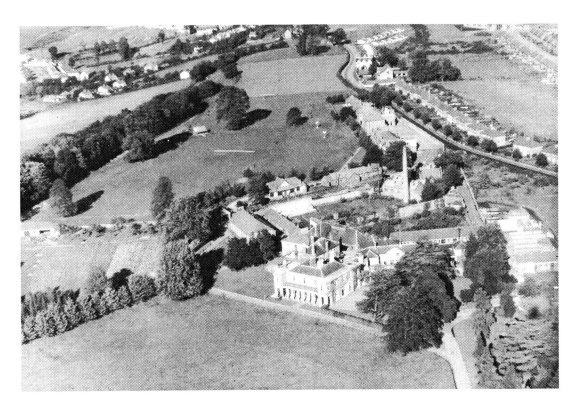

Figure 7.3: Brentry from the air, 14 September 1954

trespassers but also a recognition of the fire risk of having wards locked with no staff present to unlock them. Staff were able to 'discipline' and sanction the patients without obtaining the prior permission of the medical staff by doing such things as stopping cigarettes or not allowing trips to see the film being shown in the hall. All the patients smoked, and at times of celebration such as sports days staff would carry around cigarettes for distribution. There were a lot of minor rules that the patients had to learn though, such as the dangers of the Chief Male Nurse seeing you walk on the grass!

Patients rose as the day staff came on at 7.30am and had breakfast at 8am. Many would be bathed after breakfast, or the staff would go with them to their activities. Lunch was on the ward at 12.00 and then more activity occurred, including the afternoon social events. Tea was at 5pm and then the patients would drift to bed. All of the less able and many of the more able were in bed by the time the night staff arrived at 7.30pm.

Haig was used as a locked ward for the "repeated absconders" where up to 15 patients were continuously supervised as the "Special Party". This was the ward where the straight-jacket was most likely to be used. The group was not however supervised in the dormitory which once enabled a group to escape out of the window using bed sheets whilst a man stood behind the door to knock out the night nurse if he opened the door when doing his rounds. They were recaptured.[13]

The Board of Control continued to visit under the new NHS and the inspectors continued to press for the House Committee to further improve conditions. They recommended the provision of indoor slippers for the patients and complained that the more able patients had to go to bed at 7.30pm, before the night staff came on duty. The House Committee appear to been happy with Dr Mason's explanation that only the 'low grades' were put to bed at 7.30pm whilst the 'high grade' patients went to bed at the 'late' hour of 9pm.[14]

One of the changes brought about by the inclusion of Brentry within the NHS was that Brentry started to emulate Hortham by keeping its files on patients on the wards. Up to this date few records had been kept. The main records kept had been the legal documents about detention, held in the central offices. This can be seen as symptomatic of the patients being turned into subjects of medical care and study, rather than social care. Part of this medical drive was due to the colonies now being managed by RHBs who mainly managed acute hospitals. One example of this was a common view by managers that patients should not be allowed to work. This was because of their experiences in acute hospitals that inpatients were too ill to work.[15] The result was a growing reluctance over the first 30 years of the NHS for the patients to be employed about the hospitals, unless it was specifically for 'therapy'. Initially after the war the patients were not paid any money for their work but were paid in tokens. This was changed to money as the risk of absconding diminished.

After 1948 there were virtually no other residential facilities for people with 'mental deficiency' at that time so hospitals continued to act as social care residences. Hortham took all the admissions from the community and patients were in general now admitted to Brentry from Hortham and the other ancillary hostels. However as there was always a dire shortage of beds some people were always of necessity admitted directly from the community to Brentry. The people being admitted were now coming from the Bristol area and were not the trouble-makers being sent a long distance away to Bristol. It now admitted a greater range of abilities with more less able people reaching Brentry. The number of admissions probably went up after 1952 when the Minister recognised the lack of alternative and directed the mental deficiency hospitals to admit patients for short periods without legal formality. The "Circular 5/52" patients became the short term assessment and respite care admissions of the next few years with most using Hortham.

The discharge and lack of admission of more able patients should be seen in the context of the new economic situation of the country. There was little unemployment so there was some hope of employment for the most able. The post-war building boom had demolished many of the old slums and made it easier for families to meet the physical housing requirements for people to be returned to them. Child benefit, national insurance and national assistance from the National Assistance Board made it financially more feasible for people to be cared for by their families. Now people tended to leave their families because their parents could not physically care for them alongside their other children, rather than because of poor housing or poverty.

Despite the addition of several hostels in Bristol and Bath to the group Brentry House Committee decided to pursue the idea of developing a hostel for Brentry and to this end negotiated for the purchase of "The Wyck" from Bristol Corporation. However the renovation costs proved too high so the purchase was dropped. Instead the Committee recommended that they be allowed to purchase an acre of land nearby and build some pre-fabricated buildings on it for a hostel for 24 patients alongside the building of a Nurses' School.[16] This never happened and the plan was not pursued further. At the same meeting in 1949 the committee recognised the terrible state of Kipling Ward and recommended the building of a new ward for 40 patients to replace it. However this did not happen for another 20 years. Only the vital building tasks occurred such as the sealing of the old deep well which had supplied the original colony[17] and the repair of the chapel which was badly damaged in the air-raids.[18] However at the end of the 1950s the pressure for ground floor beds forced the division of Jellicoe into two extended flats – a ground floor Baldwin and top floor Jellicoe. The exact date of this conversion is unknown but it was probably done between 1955 and 1966.[19]

The problem with all these recommendations to buy land and build hostels, schools and wards was that the House Committee had lost its power over capital projects. All of these recommendations had to pass through the Hortham-Brentry Hospital Management Committee to the Regional Hospital Board who would balance its request against those of the acute hospitals and the restrictions of the national bankruptcy. The RHB's wider priorities did not always coincide with those of the patients of Brentry. For example the RHB quickly approved the building of a building to act as a Nurses lecture theatre, staff refectory and visitors waiting room.[20] It thus improved recruitment and training but it refused for almost 20 years to replace the ward buildings despite the House Committee identifying them as slums.

The replacements came only when national and local scandals changed the priorities of the Ministry and RHB.

John Straffen

One person outside of Brentry who affected its relationship with the public was the high profile trials of John Straffen in 1951 and 1952 for the murder of young girls. He was once an inpatient at Hortham and his trial and conviction sent shock waves across the system and led to many groups closing their facilities to the residents of Mental Deficiency hospitals. His trial has been the subject of at least one book[21] and he has been featured in films on serial killers. He is currently (January 2002) the longest serving prisoner in England.

John Thomas Straffen was born in Hampshire in 1930.[22] His father was in the army and at the age of two John travelled to India with his parents to return at the age of 8 to Bath where he went to an ordinary school. At the age of nine he was charged with the theft of a purse from a girl and was placed on probation. His probation officer later recalled that he was one of 6 children with four younger sisters. He responded to the work of the probation officer: 'let there be no mistake about that. John really tried to become a good boy.'[23] However he then fell into 'bad company'. A year later he reappeared in court for breaching his probation order, was certified as a 'mental defective' and sent to St Joseph's Home, Sambourne, Warwickshire, and then to Besford Court, Worcester, from where he was discharged on reaching the age of 16. He returned to Bath and worked as an errand boy. Twelve months later he was charged with housebreaking and committed as an adult mental defective. He was not sent to prison despite additional concerns: he asked for 13 other similar charges to be taken into account; he was said to have also killed five fowl by wringing their necks; the police had twice received complaints that he had placed his hand over the mouth of girls who were strangers to him. To one he had said "What would you do if I killed you? I have done it before." The girls escaped uninjured but John later told the police he had committed a number of sexual offences, though they could find no evidence of this. He was sent to Hortham on the 10 October 1947 under section 8 of the Mental Deficiency Act (as a person convicted of a criminal offence). Here he absconded a few times but worked at a hostel and on licence a few times before being discharged on licence to his mother in April 1951. At this time he was seen as a simple, easily led lad who could not read words longer than 3 letters.

Whilst Straffen was at Bath two girls were murdered on the 15th July and 8th August 1951.

> Bath police announced late tonight that John Thomas Straffen, 21, single, a labourer, Fountain-buildings, Bath has been charged with the murder of Cicely Batstone, nine, who was found dead in a field here at 8.30am to-day....Cicely's home in Camden-road, Bath, is a short distance from the copse where Brenda Goddard, six, was found strangled nearly a month ago.[24]

John was put up for trial at Taunton Assizes in October 1951. John revealed at the trial that he had met Cicely at the cinema and walked together before he strangled her. However the jury found him unfit to plead after the judge instructed them that to try him would be like trying a little child. The consequence of this was that he was sent to Broadmoor.[25]

John escaped from Broadmoor for four hours on the 29th April 1952. Shortly after his recapture the body of Linda Bowyer, aged 5, was found strangled at Farley Hill, Berkshire, where he had been caught. He was charged with the murder and tried at Winchester Assizes on July 23rd. Much of the trial seems to have centred on whether or not he was responsible enough to be convicted. It was held that his mental defectiveness and his mental age of 9½ years did not in itself make him insane to the point that he was not guilty. It is noteworthy that at an early stage the jury were told of the past deaths for which he had not been formally convicted as well as the burglaries for which he had been convicted as a child.[26] Reading the newspaper accounts it is easy to conclude that the jury were being asked to ensure that his past strangulations be avenged even though the jury were reminded that they were only trying

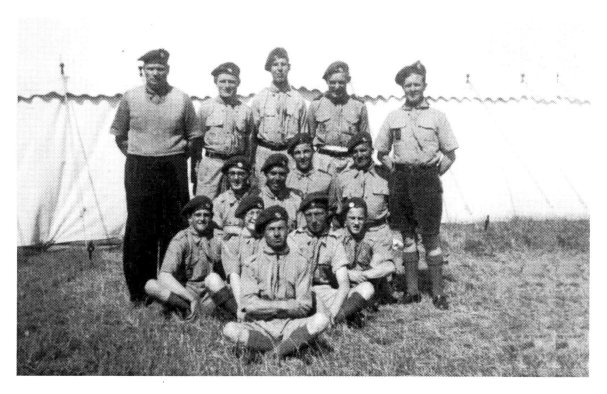

Figure 7.4: Scout Group at Brean Down, about 1957. In the back row, Mr George, scout master is on left and Mr Phillips, assistant scout master, is on right.

him for the death of Linda. The jury took only 29 minutes to find him guilty. This was so fast that it took another 24 minutes to get the judge back from lunch to hear their verdict. He sentenced John to hang.[27]

The appeal was dismissed in August but he was however reprieved on the 29th August,[28] sentenced to life imprisonment and returned to Broadmoor. It was pointed out that the trial had become preoccupied with the discussion of whether or not he was insane rather than if he was not intelligent enough to instruct his defence and therefore to be tried.[29] As the medico-legal correspondent wrote for the British Medical Journal:

> Let it be conceded that it is in the interest of the community that Straffen should be conclusively prevented from adding to the terrible toll he has taken of little girls in his dislike for the police; it yet remains difficult in the light of the facts to reconcile the course of his first trial with the course of the second. People may well think that this was not one of the clearest examples of the administration of justice.[30]

John Straffen's murder of three girls had several severe repercussions. Not only were the public more wary of the inmates of Brentry but people were now more cautious of sending patients out on licence as it was when on licence that John had committed his first two murders.

Recreation

After a 9 year absence the Scout Group was reformed in 1952 under Mr Smailes, Assistant Chief Nurse, as the 114th Bristol. This was quite an achievement, as in the previous years many of the more able and suitable patients had been discharged or sent out on licence. At first two patrols were run as occurred previously but this soon shrank to one due to a lack of cadets. The Scout Group at first held a summer camp at Cranham Woods with other scout troops where they are said to have stood out due to their adult age. They were not allowed to go again as soon afterwards there was a complaint from the:

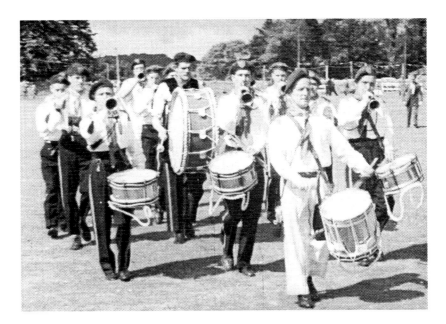

Figure 7.5: The scout band on Open Day.

> Parish Counsellors of Cranham. The Chairman of the Council stated that parishioners had said they hoped no more Scouts would be coming there to Camp from Mental Deficiency Colonies. There was no complaint against the Scouts themselves, but the request was made following the publicity given in the national newspapers to the actions of a certain mental defective who was tried on a serious charge [John Straffen].[31]

After this the weekend and annual camps were curtailed for a time due to a lack of equipment and sites. After Mr Smailes's retirement in 1955 (after 36 years service) Staff Nurse Prosser became scout master, then Charge Nurse George. For a time the scout camps had to all be held on the Brentry site, but in 1956 a summer camp started to be held at Brean (Figure 7.4). The troop only lasted for a few more years before being finally disbanded, but it also formed the core of a drum and bugle band that would entertain the visitors and residents on Open Days (Figure 7.5). In addition for a few years about five or seven of the scouts would work on an army camp for a week or two, washing up and cleaning whilst supervised by the scout master.

However public fears about the patients were being reinforced by managers who implied that they were mentally ill rather than mentally defective. When the local Girl Guides applied to camp in the woods by Berwick Lodge they were informed:

> Berwick Lodge is an ancillary unit of a psychiatric hospital; and … Girl Guides should not be allowed to wander about within the precincts of Berwick Lodge unless accompanied by a responsible adult.[32]

By now Brentry had a long tradition of running a Cricket and Football teams both of which generally did well with the football team (Figure 7.6) reaching Division II of the Church of England League in 1952. However the shallow soil on the upper recreation ground prevented any natural pitch from lasting for any length of time, so in 1950 the cricket wicket was laid to concrete with a matting pitch laid on top. Football matches were played on Thursdays and Saturdays. For all the sport being played with outside teams though, there was only a shed to change in, unlike the sports pavilion Hortham had, so visiting teams would usually change and bathe on Shackleton and have their tea in the staff mess.[33] Dr Heaton-Ward founded a rugby team (Figure 7.7) at Brentry. He recalls that:

> I started the only admittedly mentally handicapped rugger team in Bristol, if not in the country! As Brentry Hospital had a long soccer tradition, we had to overcome a certain amount of opposition and it was made very clear that we

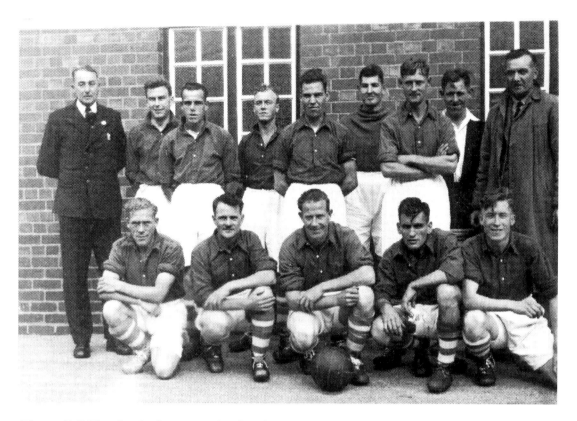

Figure 7.6 The football team at its first league game on 9 Oct 1951 - Brentry Colony v Ashton Vale - Brentry won 2-1

Back Row: Mr Wagland [charge nurse]; Mr Brackenburn; L Gould; O Gould; T Richards; J Knight; G Brewin; L Buckle; Mr Flook [deputy head nurse].
Front row: Powell; Mr Dagger [head nurse]; W Harding; Mr Wood [engineer]; R Noyes

were not to poach players from the soccer team. This meant we ended up with a team consisting of about five members of staff and ten members of the "special party". These were patients with borderline handicap, who were habitual absconders, subjected to close supervision in a locked ward, and who regarded themselves in many ways as outlawed from the rest of the hospital. However, once they became members of the hospital rugger team, they felt less outcast and a pride in representing the hospital. It did not stop them absconding, but they never let the team down by doing so when playing in away matches, neither did it stop them delighting in tackling with considerable ferocity members of staff, particularly the Deputy Medical Superintendent, during preseason trial games![34]

In time the number of residents able enough to be players dwindled and the football and rugby teams came to interchange players to help each other out. By the mid 1950s it was becoming difficult to field teams and the football team withdrew from the league for a year, re-entering in the lower, third division. The rugby team was terminated at the end of the season in 1954, after the loss of Dr Heaton-Ward who left to become Medical Superintendent of the Stoke Park Group. It had however already failed to raise a team for several matches during the season. By 1958 the Football team was managing very few matches with outside teams and the team wound up soon afterwards as a formal league side but matches were still played, mainly between hospitals, but also with some of the local businesses or police.

In the 1950s televisions made an appearance and started to oust the billiard table as the main entertainment for the residents. Initially they only appeared in the patients' social club but they spread around the wards after a few years. Colour televisions made their appearance in the 1970s. Weekly films came to be shown in the concert hall.

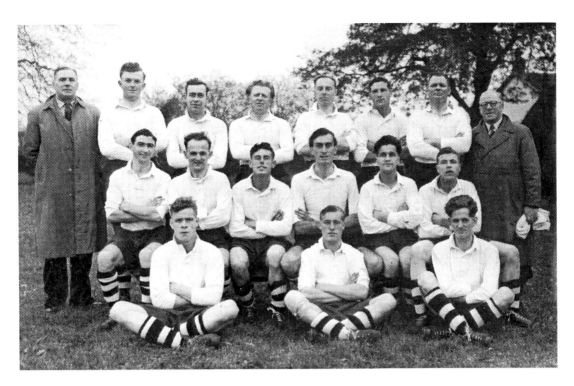

Figure 7.7: Brentry Hospital RFC. 1951-2

Back Row: Mr R Musker (Chairman and charge nurse); Mr Bishop; Mr Moore; Mr O Smith; Mr Williams; J Sandalls; Mr George; Mr H Baldwin (Hon. Sec.)
Middle row: Mr Jones; Mr Lear; H Bexton; Dr Heaton Ward (Captain); P Miller; C Robins
Front: G Howard; J Dunn; Mr P Roberts

The patients of Hortham and Brentry were eventually encouraged to mix, with a small number of each being bussed over to the other site for monthly dances. In addition the Hortham Guides would perform dances at the Brentry Sports Day and took over from the men the task of making the teas for the visitors. A small group of Brentry men went to Hortham to learn dancing with the Hortham women.[35]

The Sports Day was held annually in mid summer and always seemed to have sunny weather (Figures 7.8 and 7.9). In 1954 the 'H.W.Cornish Cup' was created from a spontaneous collection made by the residents for a wreath for Mr Cornish who died on the 31st December 1953 after having worked at Brentry as Tailor since 1935. His widow did not want any flowers so the money was used to buy the solid silver cup in memory of his keen interest in sport. In 1955 the Sports Day started to include inter-hospital competitions, with teams from Cambridge House (Farleigh) and Hortham attending. Links with Cambridge House had already been strengthened by the Nurses School expanding to include it.

There was not much contact with the community initially. The hospital had fewer walls and fences around the villas. Neighbours of the period recall that the 'Brentry lads' would often wander out of the grounds and around the neighbouring streets and the children of the neighbourhood were warned by their parents to 'be careful' with them, especially after John Straffen. Many of the less able would wander off site and have to be chased and called back not because they were purposefully escaping but because they had not realised the boundaries of the site. The lowest level of parole consisted of a group of 'lads' walking in file with a member of staff at each end. This could progress to solo parole, but some residents pre-empted this by absconding when working on the neighbouring fields. The police would usually be able to find them as the institutional clothing always helped to identify the escapees.

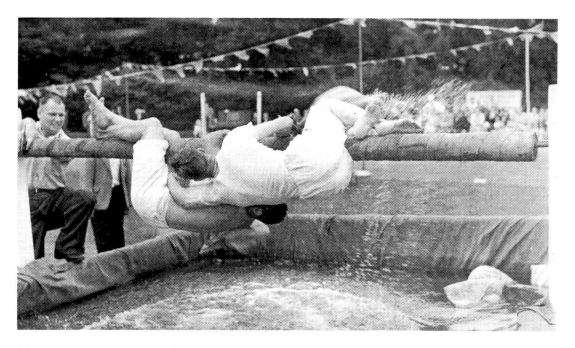

Figure 7.8: Sports day 1952

Work

Immediately after the war many of the patients used to work on the Brentry gardens and the houses in the neighbourhood could ask for 'boys' to be sent to do their gardens for them.[36] However the numbers able to do this dropped and by 1951 there were not enough patients at Brentry able enough to maintain the gardens. The ornamental gardens around the main house suffered and were moved to a style that needed less maintenance (Figure 7.10). The demise of the farm at Brentry was further hastened by the Government's shortage of money. In the 1950s the Ministry of Health wanted Hospitals to sell any 'surplus' land to raise capital. As a result in 1957 Brentry got rid of part of its remaining 50 acres of land. The pigs and cattle whose pedigrees had been so carefully recorded and which were the most profitable part of the farm, had to be sold and the farm work limited to market gardening. Despite the re-use of the field in front of the main house as a potato field the farm and land work now started to be unprofitable for the first time. In addition the higher skills demanded by the farmers outside and the reduced ability levels of the men admitted meant that the farming 'trainees' needed more supervision and were less able to work towards leaving to work on outside farms. Work became more obviously one of supplying food to the hospital rather than that of training to become a modern farm labourer. All the mental deficiency hospitals of the area had the same problems of reduced capacity to operate farms and train patients to be farm workers. The 'No. 2 Land Party' (the 'special party' from Haig) were taken in an escorted group to work in the fields – and the group had to be found new work as the field work folded. However this was not unpopular in the hospital as the field work had come to be seen as punishment by most of the patients and also by the staff who had to escort and work alongside them.

The farm was slowly eroded to nothing - in 1960 the management committee asked the Medical Superintendent to somehow make more patients available to work on the farm.[37] Later the same year the land being cultivated was still too much for the patients currently available and it was decided to put 15 acres by the lower village down to grass.[38] Another 5 acres by it was given up in 1963 as it was not felt to be worthwhile purchasing new machinery to utilise it.[39]

The loss of the farm buildings was completed in 1965 when the Farm buildings were converted into an 'Industrial Therapy' Unit.[40] Thirty acres were leased out for some time, but eventually the House Committee recommended that they be sold, though the Regional Board resisted this for a time.[41]

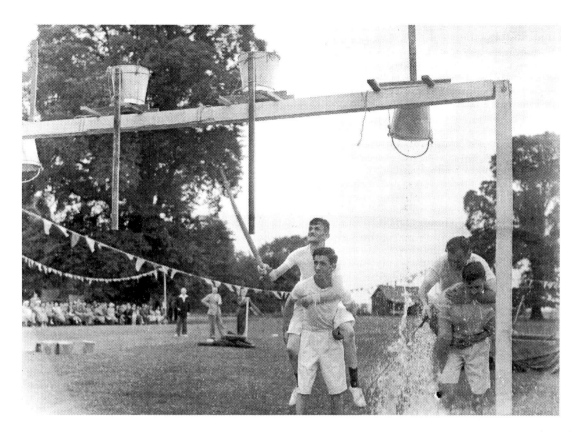

Figure 7.9: Sports Day 1952

The loss of farming did not just apply to Brentry. The hospital group operated the two agricultural hostels at Newent and Shurdlington in Gloucestershire. With the loss of work there Newent closed in 1954. By the end of the 1950s many of the residents at Shurdlington were unemployed and it was decided after discussions to move it nearer Bristol so the men were able to work in Bristol as well as in local farms. Berwick Lodge was purchased and the first patients moved in with their warden in January 1959 and Shurdlington closed that year.

Immediately after the War, patients were going out on licence either on day parole to work or for protracted periods prior to discharge. There was then a change in the system of supervision. The National Association for Mental Health was the supervisor, but after the NHS started they started levying fees to do this so it was decided to make this supervision the task of the local authorities. As a result supervision became less reliable, especially when patients were sent on licence away from their responsible authority. In 1951 there were still almost 70 people, or a sixth of the hospital, out on licence. Two years later the superintendent reported that all patients suitable for licence had either been discharged, sent to hostels or were out on private licence so few were now sent out on daily licence from Brentry.[42] From this time only about 20 patients were being sent out on leave at any one time. Brentry was becoming more isolated from the local working community.

The loss of farming as an occupation was coupled with the loss of the Industrial Unit, which closed during the 1950s due to the lack of suitable men. Similarly the old practice of using patients overtly to help with building work, painting and labouring declined. Now the patients did 'Occupational Therapy', which for the more able still comprised helping out the staff washing floors or working in the boot and mattress shop, the tailors or sewing rooms, the laundry or the kitchen, to help maintain the hospital.[43] This brought the hospital into line with the acute hospitals with no patient working, but doing "therapy". The tasks expected of them though were less than before.

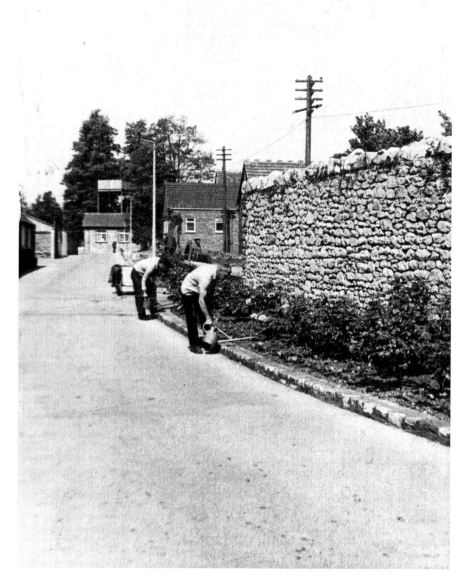

Figure 7.10 Gardening by Dickens, late 1960s. Much of the wall in the foreground had been demolished, but it is part of the wall and fence that surrounded the blocks.

Many of the activities to be called Occupational Therapy appear to have been happening before the war as the occupations cited in 1932 included basket, fine leather and raffia work (see page 67). Occupational Therapy itself is first formally discussed in 1953 when the service acquired 'materials ... to do the simplest forms of Occupational Therapy'.[44] It was also hoped 'to restore the Occupational Therapy departments to their former true purpose of occupying and teaching patients rather than that of purely commercial concern'. As the decade progressed the Occupational Therapy department came to provide more in the way of rug and basket making.[45] Some of these articles were displayed in the 1955 and 1956 British Handicrafts Exhibitions.[46] The 'Occupational Therapists' were not qualified but the activities were carried out by nurses and trainers – again the name had changed but not much of the activity. The ward nurses still continued onto the therapy units to work with the patients there and had no extra training for the task, though some nurses were specified as having a lead in running the therapy units.

Some special party 'boys'

The clinical notes of the inmates at Brentry discharged prior to 1970 are now being destroyed by the Bath and North East Somerset Primary Care Trust, who currently cares for them. However a dip into the records of some of those who recurrently absconded, illustrates the lives of the more able there. Here are modified accounts of three of the 'boys' on the 'special party', whose records no longer exist.[47]

Barry was the youngest of three brothers. He grew up on the coast of Essex and went to a special school there where he made 'little progress' and 'had no initiative'. At the age of 14 schooling stopped and he was left at home, with nothing to do and his parents both working. After a few months he was twice convicted of stealing and was sent to Stoke Park at the age of 15. At 16 he was sent back to a mental deficiency colony near his parents. They wanted him home but their house was now felt to be too small to accommodate him. His father offered to get him a job alongside him as a labourer but this was not permitted.

In 1949, at the age of 18, he was transferred to Brentry in exchange for another patient whose family wanted him in Essex. By now Barry's mother was dead and his father was over 60. At this time Barry is described as 'a feeble minded man who looks less than his life age and reacts to questions about himself with childish loquacity. He assures me of his future good conduct. He has the mental age of an eight year old'.

At Brentry Barry immediately asked to be returned to be near his home and for the next few years was clearly worried that he had not heard from his family. Attempts by the hospital to contact his father failed as his father moved and could not be traced despite attempts to do so. Barry later asked to be transferred to South London to be nearer his brother, but was told that this was not possible as his brother had shown no interest in him. Barry moved through several wards at Brentry and often complained of being teased or bullied by others. He worked in the Kitchens and then later on Kipling Lodge, and is usually reported as a cheerful and good worker. However he regularly absconded. After doing so he was usually placed on 'No.2 Party, Haig Lodge' [the 'special' party] for 3 months. He did however, manage to escape from the special party whilst working in the lower field. He continued to abscond both from the Special Party and from other Lodges for the next few years, until by 1956 he was absconding only once a year and was seen as being generally well behaved. He was usually caught close to Brentry, but he sometimes made it to Essex before he was returned. In 1958 he was felt to be well enough behaved to be granted parole to leave the grounds, but he still absconded about once a year. He was made a voluntary patient under the 1959 Mental Health Act and soon afterwards left without warning and returned to his home town where he later was found living with his father and working in a hotel.

Bill came to Brentry after a long and hard life. He had been a vagrant who travelled around England and had a long list of convictions for assault (on policemen) and drunkenness. At the age of 43 he was sent to a Workhouse Institution where he was aggressive and escaped, so he was sent to Rampton. There he became depressed but improved and after 20 years he was sent to Brentry in 1959, to be near his relatives and in exchange for another patient who needed to be transferred to Rampton. By now he was over 60, with bouts of depression and a liking to be left alone. He was seen as amenable and co-operative, with the mental age of an eight year old.

At Brentry he was 'civil and co-operative in every way', working well as a domestic on the wards. He soon absconded and after three absences was placed on the 'Special Party'. After the 1959 Mental Health Act he was made informal, and immediately left, but a few days later readmitted himself in a destitute state. A fortnight later he was re-detained because he had been unable to look after himself when out. He then absconded 5 times in the next two years. He was transferred to Berwick Lodge, but disliked it there and returned to Brentry at his request. He was again made a voluntary patient and after leaving and returning 3 times he left for good in 1966.

When Bill absconded he seems to have travelled rough around the country, doing odd jobs and getting drunk. When he was picked up by the police he would agree to voluntarily return to Brentry rather than be charged.

Mike was born in an agricultural village just prior to the war and was first seen as 'well behaved, with a nice disposition and clean habits'. He is said to have been very aware that his mother was 'less intelligent then him', though he himself went to a special school. At the end of school he is described as 'rather arrogant and likely to get into trouble'. He was put to work on a farm but was soon dismissed for sleeping at work. He was then tried at various labouring jobs, which he attended patchily. A few months later he was convicted of burglary in the company of a known criminal, and then of assaulting a policeman when drunk. He was placed on a probation order and attempts were made to force him to move away from his parents, as the living conditions were felt to be 'appalling'. He again stole and at the age of 19 he was sent to Brentry by a court in 1960. He was found to be of low normal intelligence. He absconded five times in the first six months, once stealing a bicycle to help his escape. He also broke into the Social Club to steal beer. As a result he was placed on the 'Special Party' for a few months. He continued to escape. When returned he was fined up to 4 weeks pocket-money and sometimes was 'put to bed at weekends'. He went to work in the workshops and was allowed parole – going out accompanied by another patient. After having been in Brentry for less than 2 years he was sent on licence to live with his stepfather. He tried a series of jobs before saying he would become a farm labourer. He said he planned to marry his local girlfriend and was immediately asked to return to Brentry to see the doctor. Not knowing why, he immediately married his girl before going to Brentry. He was allowed to stay out on leave 'under the considerable influence of his wife', living in very simple accommodation, cooking on the open fire. After a year he became unemployed after an injury. He then lived with his wife in a home rented by his father-in-law who complained that Mike was not signing on, but living on his goodwill. However as he had been out for 6 months he was formally discharged from Brentry and we hear no more of him.

Notes

[1] This part is based on the account given by Charles Webster, in *The Health Services since the War: Volume 1 - Problems of health care, the National Health Service before 1957.* H.M.S.O. 1988. Particularly pages 326ff

[2] see Historical Section of Royal Commission on Law relating to Mental Illness and Mental Deficiency 1957 and K. Jones: *Asylums and After.*

[3] For details see P K Carpenter: The Georgian Idiot Hospital at Bath. *History of Psychiatry* 1998. **9:**471-89 and P K Carpenter: The Bath Idiot and Imbecile Institution. *History of Psychiatry* 2000. **11:**163-88.

[4] *BRO:* Brentry House Committee 15 Sept 1949

[5] 6th annual report of Hortham-Brentry H.M.C.

[6] Brentry House Committee 20 Jan 1949 Item 6(a)

[7] 2nd annual report

[8] 2nd annual report

[9] 4th annual report

10 5th annual report

[10] 5th annual report
[11] 8th annual report. Howse was appointed Group Secretary in 1955. The previous group secretary, Mr Fellows, had been working at Hortham since it first opened in 1932.
[12] *Bristol Evening Post* Dec 10th 1955.
[13] Reminiscence J Phillips
[14] Brentry House Committee 21 July 1949
[15] Personal comments of a doctor who was on the committee.
[16] Brentry House Committee 19 June 1949
[17] Brentry House Committee 13 Oct 1949
[18] 2nd annual report
[19] Judging from the list of wards in 1966. Staff starting in 1969 do not recall it being one ward. Staff starting in 1955 recall its division but cannot date it.
[20] Brentry House Committee 13 Oct 1949
[21] *The Trial of John Thomas Straffen.* (ed: Letitia Fairfield and Fullbrook.) London and Edinburgh: Hodge, 1954.
[22] *Ibid*, see also newspaper articles of trial, eg. *Bristol Evening World* 23 July 1952, page 3
[23] *Empire News*, 27 July 1952.
[24] *Bristol Evening World*, 8 August 1951.
[25] *British Medical Journal* 6 September 1952, pages 568-9.
[26] See *Lancet* August 2nd 1952 page 239.
[27] See for example *News of the World* 27 July 1952, page 3
[28] *The Times* 1 September 1952
[29] see letter of Russell Brain, *The Times*, 1 September 1952, page 5.
[30] *British Medical Journal* 6 September 1952, page 569
[31] 4th annual report - report for Hortham (see also scout report for Brentry)
[32] Hortham/Brentry Committee May 1960 Min. 11
[33] H.M.C. Finance Committee Sept 1973 Minute 52, and memories Jim Telling
[34] A Heaton-Ward; 'Perspective'. *Psychiatric Bulletin* (1989) **13**:225-30, page 227.
[35] 5th annual report
[36] Personal reminiscence of neighbour who is a doctor
[37] Hortham/Brentry Committee May 1960 Minute 8.
[38] Hortham/Brentry Committee 27 Sept 1960 Minute 30.
[39] Hortham/Brentry Committee 8 April 1963 Minute 27.
[40] Brentry House Committee 17 Dec 1965, (and 30 march 65 Min 74)
[41] Hortham/Brentry Committee 24 Sept 68, minute 30; 31 July 1969 Minute 20.
[42] 4th Annual report for 1952-3.
[43] see 5th annual report (1954)
[44] 4th annual report - Brentry
[45] 6th annual report
[46] 7th & 8th annual report
[47] These accounts are altered to remove all identifying information.

The 1959 Mental Health Act

During the 1950s the problems of the mental illness asylums and mental deficiency colonies could not be masked by the 'word magic' of renaming them hospitals and including them in the NHS. In 1954 the first parliamentary debate on mental health for 24 years was triggered when the following Private Member's Bill was introduced into the House of Commons:

> That this House, while recognising the advances made in recent years in the treatment of mental patients, expresses its concern at the serious overcrowding of mental hospitals and mental deficiency hospitals, and at the acute shortage of nursing and junior medical staff in the Mental Health Service; and calls upon HM Government and the hospital authorities to make adequate provision for the modernisation and development of this essential service.[1]

The debate highlighted the terrible state of the hospitals, but also pointed out that the new welfare system and drugs meant that the old laws on the care and treatment of the mentally ill and of mental defectives urgently needed reform. What the Board of Control had been saying for over 10 years was finally listened to and a Royal Commission was set up in 1954 on the law relating to Mental Illness and Deficiency. After it reported in 1957[2] the laws were replaced by the new Mental Health Act of 1959.[3]

This Act was a radical change from the old laws. It abolished the old Lunacy Act and Mental Deficiency Acts and brought both groups under one act. It changed the law from the purpose of custody to that of treatment. The old laws had concentrated on the need to have a judicial process of commitment to deprive a person of his liberty and have the public authorities pay for him to be treated in a mental hospital or mental deficiency colony. Now the law assumed that treatment was free and that people would want to enter such hospitals. Now commitment was only necessary if the person refused treatment and where health or safety justified it. The new Act also changed the legal terms and classification of the ability levels of mental deficiency from Idiot, Imbecile and Feebleminded to Severe Subnormality and Subnormality. It also modified the category of Moral Defective to Psychopathic Disorder, which was seen as less stigmatising. In addition it prevented anyone over the age of 21 being freshly detained as having 'subnormality' or 'psychopathic disorder' unless they had been prosecuted in court for an imprisonable offence. People with 'severe subnormality' could still be detained when over the age of 21 without being charged in court. Once detained, the detention of 'minors' with 'subnormality' or 'psychopathic disorder' could be renewed until the age of 25 on the grounds of the patient's "health, safety or the protection of others", after which the medical officer could only continue renewals on the grounds of dangerousness. Of course the patient could always continue as an 'informal', or voluntary inpatient once discharged from detention.

In general the Act tried to turn the social conditions of mental deficiency and lunacy into the medical conditions of subnormality and mental illness, to be treated in the same manner as other medical conditions. The homes and hospitals were to be operated under the same legislation as other general medical institutions. Like other medical hospitals, every patient had to have a doctor who was in charge of them – a responsible medical officer [RMO]. The legislation forced the discharge of all the more able adults with mental subnormality and thus speeded the process of emptying the old mental deficiency colonies of the more able residents, though they were soon refilled by less able people as there was still no alternative accommodation. Under the old legislation the renewal of detention and act of discharge were made by the managers of the hospital, but it was now a decision made by the patient's doctor.

Medical staff changes after 1959

The new Mental Health Act passed in 1959 forced another change in Brentry Hospital. All of the long-stay people in Brentry were detained. Under the old Mental Deficiency Acts, all detained patients are reviewed and their detention renewed by the Board of Control after receiving a report from the 'visitors' of the institution, with a short medical report from 'the medical officer of the Institution'. Renewal was a legal process that did not specify the expertise of the doctor who examined the patient. This was because there were few experienced doctors at the start of the act. The new Mental Health Act assumed every inpatient had a RMO who was in charge of their treatment. As the reason for being in hospital was treatment it was now the RMO who would decide when to discharge them without reference to any committee. The RMO had to renew this detention at 6 months and then every two years after the first year of detention. During the1959 Act's introduction period the RMO had to examine all the adults in his hospital to determine if they were 'severely subnormal' (and able to be detained) or only 'subnormal'. If 'subnormal' a patient could only be detained if they had been charged with an imprisonable offence and were dangerous. He then had to decide whether or not to renew the detention if it was permissible.

With the new Act, Dr Lumsden Walker's title was changed from that of Medical Superintendent to Consultant, using the term that applied in general medical hospitals for the doctor with ultimate responsibility for patients under the care of his medical team. He was the sole Consultant for the group. The two Senior Hospital Medical Officers [SHMO], Drs Woods[4] and Leahy were not appointed consultants (in part as SHMO posts occurred in general medical hospitals separate to consultants) but they still were appointed RMOs. The Regional Hospital Board objected to this saying that only consultants could be RMOs but the Management Board pointed out that this would make Dr Walker RMO for 1400 patients which was clearly not reasonable.[5] They recommended appointing a second Consultant. The Regional Hospital Board, agreed as an emergency measure to appoint a second consultant shared with Stoke Park. Dr Jancar was appointed to this post on 1 March 1962.[6] The Management Committee said its long term plan was to change the two SHMO posts into consultant posts. In the meantime it decided that the contracts of the SHMOs, which stated that they were to have 'continuous clinical responsibility for patients', meant that they fitted the Regional Board's requirement that RMOs had 'ultimate clinical responsibility'. As a result they could, and did appoint Drs Woods and Leahy as RMOs under the 1959 Act.[7] This was a creative interpretation as the SHMOs were responsible to consultants and were not independent in the manner of RMOs who were said to be 'answerable to no other doctor for determining the medical care of a patient' – the doctor with ultimate responsibility.

The effect of the Act was that Dr Walker had to review with the SHMOs all the patients on the wards. All 1400 had to be assessed to determine if they met the criteria for Subnormality or Severe Subnormality and if they should be discharged under the new Act to remain as informal patients. The task was enormous. By 1965 almost 90% of the inpatients at Hortham were discharged to informal status but the process was much slower at Brentry. Here the main medical officer was Dr Leahy who did not work at Hortham. The staff at Brentry appear to have found it difficult to justify discharging patients from detention.

When Dr Grace Woods left Hortham in 1965 her post was replaced by a new consultant post, filled by Dr Fairburn[8] which helped the staffing position and RMO status at Hortham but not at Brentry where the fudging of the RMO status of Dr Leahy had repercussions as Dr Leahy tried to establish if he was a consultant or not. For example in 1966 the Regional Board stated that consultants had final responsibility for treatments and should therefore control admissions. Dr Leahy protested that as RMO he controlled admissions and treatments. The Management Board avoided the issue by referring the matter to the RHB and stating that consultants could delegate their admission rights to SHMOs.[9] The next year, when Dr Gordon Russell was appointed consultant it was specifically stated that he would have 'overall responsibility' for Dr Leahy's beds.[10]

Dr Leahy appears to have had many disputes with the management as the hospital management committee refer to them several times. In addition there are stories of his disputes with other staff within the system. His 'mistreatment' over the fudged RMO status must have embittered him over other issues, and much of the minutes seem to be about him being told to do things that he did not want to do. The management disputes recorded were usually about his status as RMO but in addition he was given formal notice to quit his flat[11] at Brentry in 1962 after he refused to move out of it. His was the last family to live in the main building in the accommodation first occupied by the Burdens, as it was then converted to office accommodation. The old living room was turned in to the Board Room and the Hospital Secretary took over the room opposite the top of the stairs. Staff and patients were only allowed up to this floor by invitation – they went up the stairs only if they were in trouble or applying for a job. Leahy also got into trouble with the Management Committee in 1967 for publishing a survey of Athletes Foot at Brentry without obtaining permission for either the publication or the research, though he claimed he had received permission from Dr Walker prior to his departure.[12]

In 1967 there was a change of consultants with the appointment of a new consultant and Dr Gordon Russell becoming full time. Dr Gordon Russell took on 48 beds at Brentry, the new consultant (Dr Lower) was to have 100 and also have overall responsibility of the remainder of the beds managed by Dr Leahy.[13]

In 1970 Dr Leahy was told that he was losing his status as RMO. He objected and appealed to the Regional Hospital Board, but the Board upheld the change, which was not surprising given the board's prior insistence that only Consultants acted as RMO.[14] The new fourth consultant appointed to the group, Dr Bird, was asked to share the office of Dr Leahy when he started in April 1971.[15] It rapidly became clear that this was not a good option and within days of Dr Bird starting in post Dr Leahy was 'asked' to move out to an office in Shackleton.[16]

Nurse changes after 1959

Nursing staffing levels continued to be a problem. The main attraction to working at Brentry was the availability of houses for staff, so many of the staff recruited were married and in need of a house. However many of the staff cottages were in a poor state, to the point that in 1966 it was suggested that many were demolished, but the regional architect stated that they were sound and merited improving when money was available.[17] In 1960 it was planned to build a nurses home to attract staff but this was abandoned when Bristol Corporation allocated three council houses for the use of staff of Brentry, and offered more if needed.[18] The need for accommodation for young single nurses continued and at one point it was planned to convert the Nursing Home at Hortham to take male student nurses from Brentry.[19]

In 1962 Brentry was already using female Nursing Auxillaries on some of the wards and so was ahead of Hortham which still rigorously segregated female nurses from male patients.[20] This was probably a necessity due to the lack of recruitment of male staff. In 1963 it was again noted with regret that an increasing number of staff were having to work beyond the age of retirement[21] due to the lack of recruitment because of the thriving economy in Bristol and availability of better higher paid jobs in local industry.

Staff still worked a 4 day 12 hour long shift system. In 1964 there was a directive[22] to reduce the hours worked by four hours a fortnight. At the same time Whitley Council rules were introduced that forbade staff being paid overtime and required them to be given time off in lieu. The management team found the staffing problems magnified overnight. Now overtime could not be used to cover staff vacancies.[23] In 1967 the staff asked if they could manage the requirement for reduced hours (from 88 hours a fortnight to 84 hours) by accumulating the hours and taking a day off in lieu but were told that this would break the working hours requirement and that the 4 hour reduction would have to be covered by recruiting more staff for the evening.[24]

Deputy charge nurses were approved in 1965 to help recruitment.[25] However it was soon afterwards declared by the ministry that there could not be deputies where there were two nurse teams working opposite to each other (as occurred with the long shift) unless the Charge Nurse worked a shift that overlapped both teams.[26] The result was that eventually

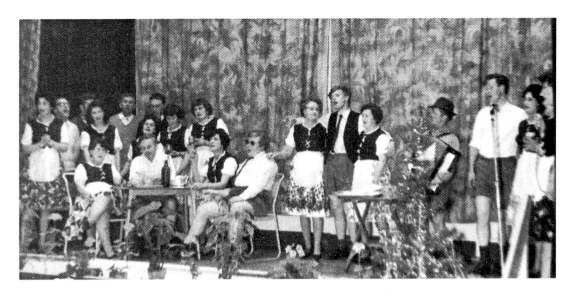

Figure 8.1: Staff performance of Sound of Music in the late 1960s

Brentry wards ran with two charge nurses for each ward - one for each nursing team. It was now even more difficult to ensure that patients were treated consistently by all the staff.

In 1971 another attempt was made to bring in a revised shift system when the Hospital Advisory Service recommended a change to a five day week shift system. However the nurses refused through their union, saying they wanted to continue with the present long shift.[27] A compromise was implemented with the agreement of COHSE whereby staff worked 2 long days and 3 short days a week.[28]

There continued to be male student nurses at Brentry as part of the nursing school of the group. In 1968 the area nurse training committee refused the recruitment of female student nurses specifically for Brentry but suggested females were recruited to the group training scheme. The local committee approved this[29] but there is not much evidence of many female students working at Brentry. The male student nurses based at Brentry did not need to spend much clinical time outside of Brentry - the only ward work away from Brentry was that with children which of necessity had to be at Hortham as did the formal teaching.[30] They did not train on the adult female wards at Hortham as male nurses were never expected to look after adult women. In common with the philosophy at the time and the difficulties of travel the student nurses were not expected to gain experience in a wide variety of hospitals and so still received a rather parochial experience of nursing at Brentry.

As staff recruitment was so difficult there was a drive to recruit from abroad, and in the late 1960s a group of nurses were brought over from Mauritius. It is said that some of them were housed in the upper corridor above the stables next to the staff dining room. In general though, with the problem recruiting staff, there was sometimes concern about the quality of staff working on site. Steps were taken to prevent criminal acts by the staff such as installing two drug cupboards on certain wards to prevent the theft of drugs on these wards, as then the night staff had access only to the drugs needed for the night.[31] Staff discipline was tight but the grounds for dismissal could be different to modern times - in the 1960s a nurse was disciplined for his behaviour after he had ignored several 'urgings to seek employment elsewhere'. At the hearing it was discovered that he had lied about his address to cover up the fact that he had moved in with a female nurse. He immediately submitted his resignation on the advice of his union officer. In 1970 a student nurse, Mr L J Sutherland, was placed on probation after pleading guilt of arson after setting fire to a mattress with bed-linen and patients' clothing. Shortly afterwards two laundry bags were set fire to on Baldwin but the culprit was not discovered.[32]

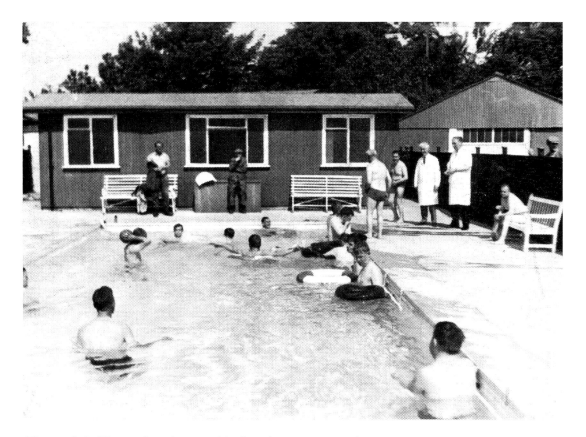

Figure 8.2: The swimming pool before it was covered.

In 1966 the unions formally protested that Brentry staff were not being short-listed for senior posts at Brentry. The Hospital Management Committee upheld the selection process, but made no comment on the success rate of Brentry staff in obtaining senior posts.[33] In the same year the Salmon Committee Report on Nursing recommended a new senior nursing structure for the whole NHS, abolishing the old post of matron. The Ministry told the regions to implement it[34], but it took over five years for the system to be introduced at Brentry and Hortham. It was only introduced after the national Hospital Advisory Service wrote a very critical report on the hospitals.[35]

Resident changes after 1959

Under the 1959 Mental Health Act adults with mild 'subnormality' could only be kept in hospital if sent there by a court of law. However few of these could be contained in an ordinary subnormality hospital. Few such places had enough staff to prevent the more able patients from absconding if they wanted to and as a result anyone who justified continued detention was usually in the special hospitals such as Rampton, either because they were violent or because they absconded. At Brentry most of the more able who remained eventually became informal patients but some remained detained against their will and this caused a problem. In 1962 the Hospital Management Committee accepted the Medical Staff Advisory Committee's recommendation to adapt a villa in the lower village for special security purposes for male patients.[36] The adaptation does not seem to have occurred though, so the need for the 'special party continued.

Like other hospitals, Brentry was overcrowded. Most of its wards were over 50 years old which compounded the problem. In 1963 Brentry officially held beds for 392 patients but actually held 444. On one ward 30 patients shared one toilet and no bathroom. That year it

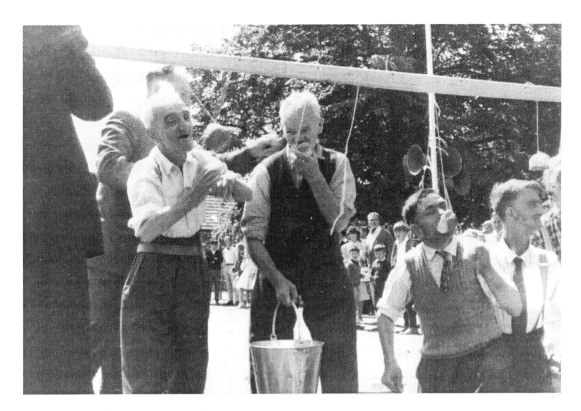

Figure 8.3: Sports day 1965

was decided that drastic action was needed and to stop all admissions to Brentry until the population fell to 420.[37]   However there was no other accommodation available in the community, so pressure for people to be admitted continued. In addition Brentry Committee itself argued that it had to admit some 'high-grade' patients to keep the hospital running.[38] Dr Leahy also refused to stop admitting patients, claiming that Brentry was not severely overcrowded.[39]   The 'ban' was formally 'postponed' in 1965 when the population reached 432.

Brentry was still a very institutional place. Patients were each supplied with three sets of clothes but these were over-washed and ill-fitting. However the appearance of the patients suffered in 1968 after a new supplies system was imposed by the RHB to reduce costs. The Hospital Management Committee expressed concern that the clothing standards be maintained as 'considerable progress has been made in eliminating the institutional appearance for patients in their clothing and introducing individuality so that they were able to mix with the community without feeling conspicuous or inferior in any way.'[40] The success of this protest is not minuted.

In 1968 Shackleton was upgraded to house 24 young male adolescents, so that the children's ward at Hortham, Lundy, could be used for the elderly.[41]   This ward was opened in the following year and accommodated 19-29 year olds with 3 monthly review of parole, privileges, occupation etc.[42]   When reviewed in 1970 it was clear that Dr Leahy was in conflict with his consultant Dr Lower who also had beds on Shackleton along with Dr Gordon Russell. All of Dr Leahy's beds on Shackleton were transferred to Dr Lower, to the displeasure of Dr Leahy who complained that he would lose contact with some patients with whom he had been associated for 15 years.[43]

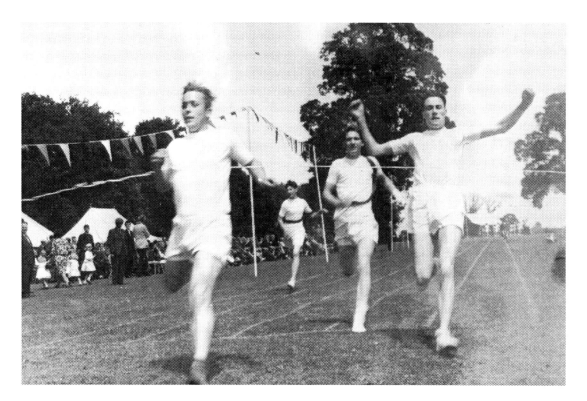

Figure 8.4: Sports day 1965

Activities

One of the main innovations of the 1960s for Brentry was the activity and contributions made by the League of Friends. It was started in 1958 to raise money for the hospital and enabled most of the new amenities that occurred at the hospital during the 1960s. In 1968 it built and donated a social club to the hospital to be used by both staff and patients. By 1969 the patients club was running a profitable shop on site for the residents and staff, though the patient's club and hall did not sell alcohol. The staff had their own social club and bar by the old original laundry buildings. Behind it was a Bowling Green mainly used by the staff and by the local community.

The provision of a swimming pool at Hortham by its League of Friends stimulated the Hospital Committee to provide Brentry with a swimming pool with the help of the League of Friends. It opened in 1967 (Figure 8.2). In 1970 there was a momentary panic when a patient, Gloria Carson, died whilst swimming at the Hortham Pool despite her being a reasonable swimmer and having two staff and four able male residents in the area. It was decided to keep the pools open. The pool was used by both staff and their families and by the patients, including those in wheelchairs. In 1971 a hard tennis court was installed by the League of Friends between the swimming pool and social club.[44]

Social activities for the male inpatients were improved in 1967 by the radical step of mixing the male and female patients of the hospital group during social events. Hortham patients and the Hillside 'girls' were taken to meet the Brentry 'boys' monthly, if only to see the films being shown every week at Brentry. They were of course heavily supervised. Horse riding started for the patients in 1971 with a weekly two hour session of pony riding using 4 ponies.[45]

Summer holidays were still very regimented with the annual sports day (Figure 8.3 and 8.4) and the mass use of a summer camp by most of the patients. In the Autumn 1972, the Bristol Children's Help Society informed the Hospital that it could no longer use their summer camp at Winscombe for patient holidays.[46] The Hospital Management Committee wrote to the RHB who were supportive of finding a holiday home within 70 miles of Bristol that could be used

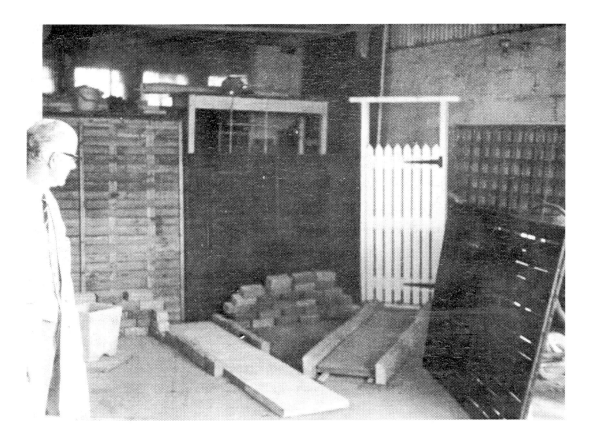

Figure 8.5: Some of the products of OT and IT in the new IT unit.

by several groups. The purchase of Boverton Camp in South Wales was entertained for some time but then abandoned due to its poor facilities though it was rented for 26 weeks for Brentry to use in 1973. One member of staff recalls the buildings there being so delapidated that the only habitable huts they found had no window openings. That holiday the patients kept out of the huts except to sleep. At the same time the Group looked at purchasing Doniford Camp, Watchet from the Ministry of Defence,[47] but this fell through and Boverton was again rented for 1974. A patient is said to have died in the abandoned swimming pool there. In the end no site was purchased and the Knoll in Clevedon was used as a holiday home.

Patient work opportunities further collapsed when the Bootshop closed in 1968. For over a year it had been running into difficulties due to the lack of suitable patients to work there. At first it was hoped that the transfer of patients from Berwick Lodge and from Hortham would improve matters[48] but this did not happen and it was decided to close the bootshop and to give the shoemaker Mr G Parry a month's notice.[49] The stock was transferred to the Bootshops at Stoke Park and Manor Park.

The Industrial Therapy Hut converted out of the piggeries was still in action, as was the concrete block unit beyond it and the new ballpoint pen assembly unit built by the swimming pool. In 1970 a new prefabricated Industrial Therapy unit was commissioned (Figure 8.5).[50] In 1971 a small fire occurred in it when someone dropped a lighted article through a broken window in the early morning. This was blamed on a patient and the staff instructed to keep the patients away from the terrapins out of hours.[51]

Notes

[1] Hansard 15 February 1954, quoted in K Jones *Asylums and After* page 148.

[2] *Report of the Royal Commission on the law relating to Mental Illness and Mental Deficiency 1954-1957.* [Cmnd.169] London: H.M.S.O., May 1957.

[3] *Mental Health Act, 1959.* (7&8 Eliz.2.Ch.72)

[4] Obituary *BMJ* 1 Jan 2000: **320** p 61

[5] Hortham/Brentry Committee Sept 1960 Minute 46 and 56.

[6] Hortham/Brentry Committee March 1961, minute 67 and 27 March 1962 minute 58.

[7] Hortham/Brentry Committee 30 May 1961 Minute 6, 29 May 1962 Minute 10

[8] Hortham/Brentry Committee 27 Jul 1965 minute 23

[9] Hortham/Brentry Committee 27 Sept 1966 Minute 30, also 29 Nov 1966 Minute 38/30

[10] Hortham/Brentry Committee31 Jan 1967 Minute 50

[11] Hortham/Brentry Committee 29 May 1962 Minute 5

[12] Hortham/Brentry Committee Special meeting 7 Sept 1967

[13] H.M.C. 28 March 1967 Min 61(50)

[14] see for example H.M.C. 28 Jan 1971.

[15] H.M.C. 28 Jan 1971 Minute 48/38

[16] H.M.C. 27 May 1971 Minute 11

[17] H.M.C. 29 Nov 1966 Min 38(34).

[18] Hortham/Brentry Committee Sept 1960 Minute 47 & 28 March 1961, Minute 67.

[19] Hortham/Brentry Committee 30 July 1968 Minute 20.

[20] Hortham/Brentry Committee 29 Main 1962 Minute 4

[21] Hortham/Brentry Committee 8 Apr 1963 Minute 16(c)

[22] HM(64)7

[23] Hortham/Brentry Committee 30 Mar 1965 Minute 75.

[24] H.M.C. 28 November 1967

[25] Hortham/Brentry Committee 27 Jul 1965 Minute 23

[26] H.M.C. 30 Nov 1965 minute 42(27)

[27] H.M.C. 21 October 1971 Minute 44/3.

[28] H.M.C. Finance Committee minutes 28 June 1972 minute 25 and 26 July 1972 Minute 33/25

[29] Hortham/Brentry Committee 28 May 1968 Minute 7

[30] memories of Brendan Sheridan

[31] H.M.C. Education Committee minutes 3 September 1970.

[32] Hortham/Brentry Committee 29 Jan 1970

[33] Hortham/Brentry Committee 24 May 1966 Minute 2

[34] HC(68)28

[35] H.M.C. 14 January 1972.

[36] Hortham/Brentry Committee 29 May 1962 Minute 21

[37] Hortham/Brentry Committee 8 Apr 1963 Minute 17

[38] Hortham/Brentry Committee 27 Jul 1965 Minute 18

[39] Hortham/Brentry Committee 28 July 1964 Minute 15(3)

[40] Hortham/Brentry Committee 24 Sept 1968 Minute 28

[41] Hortham/Brentry Committee 26 Mar 1968 Minute 68.

[42] Hortham/Brentry Committee 25 Mar 1965 Minute 56

[43] H.M.C. 29 Jan 1970 Minute 50

[44] H.M.C. Finance Committee 21 April 1971.

[45] H.M.C. 27 May 1971 Minute 6/57

[46] H.M.C. 4 August 1972 Minute 25

[47] H.M.C. 3 April 1973 minute 9

[48] H.M.C. 25 July 1967 Min 15.

[49] Finance and General Purposes Committee 16 July 1968

[50] H.M.C. 26 March 1970 minute 67.

[51] H.M.C. 1 April 1971 Minute 2

1969 and its Aftermath

Like other mental handicap hospitals Brentry reached its nadir at the end of the 1960s. As usual, money was being diverted to the high profile acute hospitals and it was a struggle to produce any improvements to the fabric of the buildings. At the same time there was little alternative accommodation and a high pressure for admissions – in the 1970s the *urgent* waiting list for admission to Stoke Park is said to have been over 2,500 (larger than the population of Stoke Park).[1] During this decade the role of the Mental Handicap hospitals (as they were being called) was being questioned but few articles appeared in the national press and the matter was largely ignored as were the hospitals behind their high walls. The Devaluation of the Pound in 1968 produced further cuts as the Regional Hospital Board estimated the devaluation would cost the region £600,000 and urged yet further economies on the already under-resourced service.

Brentry was not in good shape. It was under pressure to admit even more patients. It still had wards such as Kipling with its 'bear pit' courtyard where the patients roamed in the view of the road passing by above it. The lower village still housed the less able patients and the stench on parts of the wards there could make people physically sick. In general the staffing levels remained terrible, but many staff who worked at this time in Brentry and other Mental Handicap Hospitals now look back on these days as some of the happiest in their working lives. They describe hard work but a high working morale with a strong feeling of being in a community. After that 'the atmosphere changed'.

Scandals started to attract the attention of the media. The first was that of ill-treatment at Ely Hospital in Cardiff. On the 20 August 1967 the *News of the World* published a statement by a nursing assistant at Ely, alleging that patients were beaten, their food stolen and that the senior staff ignored the abuses. The Welsh Hospital Board set up a committee of inquiry to examine the allegations. It had limited powers but met from December 1967 to February 1968. The report published in March 1969[2] agreed that there was much ill-treatment but said that 'Most (but not all) were due to the persistence of nursing methods which were old-fashioned, untutored, rough and, on some occasions, lacking in sympathy.'[3] The inquiry recommended increased resources, improved recruitment and 'a complete reconstruction of the hospital'.

One of the members of the inquiry was the Professor of Psychiatry at Bristol, Prof. Russell Davies who did not expect to have a similar scandal on his doorstep. But in December 1968 the police visited Farleigh Hospital to investigate claims of ill-treatment. As a result Farleigh and mental handicap hospitals were thrust into the faces of the public for almost two years. National newspapers reported the exhumation of bodies in July 1969, the week-long coroner's inquiry in August 1969, the magistrates trial in December, the three week trial at the Crown Courts in Spring 1970 and the conviction of three staff. In addition the Minister of Health Richard Crossman then set up a Committee of Inquiry into the events and the management of Farleigh. The newspapers reported its proceedings over three weeks of August 1970 as well as the final report published in April 1971. This was massive and shocking publicity with headlines such as: "Patients were beaten up"[4] and "Nude patient tied up".[5] The report showed with startling openness the under-resourcing and poor state of the Mental Handicap Hospitals of the land. The inquiry criticised the long shift system and reinforced the need for the new Salmon senior nursing structure and for the mental handicap service to receive more funding. The effects of all this publicity was devastating on the staff in other mental handicap hospitals, and in Brentry there was a lot of work done by the two consultants Dr Gordon-Russell and Dr Fairburn to keep up morale despite the scandals elsewhere.

In the middle of this, Mr Crossman on the 31 October 1969 visited Stoke Park to review the situation. There he was shown the over-crowding and Dr Heaton-Ward recalls that he 'told us at the end of his visit that overcrowding was our own fault and we should refuse all admissions, even though we knew families were breaking down under the strain.'[6]

In 1969 the BBC was given permission to film in Brentry Hospital. It was for a feature on hospitals for the mentally subnormal which it was proposed to include in the programme '24 Hours'. Mrs Wilcox of the BBC stated they wanted to indicate both problems and achievements in this field. She would welcome guidance as to the most significant points. It was not intended to name or compare hospitals in the programme except that particular hospitals had particular problems and achievements. Patients would not be recognisable.[7]

The Hospital Management Committee were sufficiently impressed by the result to decide to commission a film to use in later publicity and also appointed a public relations officer. They abandoned the idea when they discovered that a 20 minute film would cost £800 – £1000.[8] By the middle of 1970 they had decided to abolish the new post of public relations officer but kept her post going[9] at the request of the Regional Hospital Board as it wanted her to act 'elsewhere in due course'. It was noted that the public relations officer had been effective in recruiting WRVS staff.[10] When she did resign in 1973, she was not replaced, on the grounds that the new voluntary organisers now did much of her work.[11] In Brentry the new co-ordinator of voluntary services was Mr T.H Malpas, who had once been the Aide-de-Camp to the Governor of Mauritius.

One of the consequences of the interest in television and filming in Brentry, was the use of Brentry as a site for filming *The White Bird*, a film starring Concorde, Alan Dobie and Stacey Tendeter, and produced by James Archibald to make money for the Duke of Edinburgh's Award Scheme.[12] This film was released in Spring 1974 and well appreciated in Bristol.

Shortly after the television programme on Brentry the Bristol Evening Post decided to campaign on its behalf. Up until then the local publicity had been directed at Farleigh and Stoke Park and the Management Committee must have been concerned that any funding directed at improving the hospitals would pass them by. The result was their co-operation with a full page article:

> Brentry Hospital, situated in 90 acres of picturesque parkland near Westbury-on-Trym, is outwardly a pleasant place. But tour some of the ward blocks built at the time of the Boer Ward, and you will find a depressing atmosphere of decay. The space is cramped, the elevation too high, and room for improvement simply does not exist.
> Take Allenby Ward, for example. The chairman of Hortham-Brentry Hospital Management Committee, Mrs. Liebe Anderson said: It ought to be gutted. It makes me shudder." Hospital group secretary Mr Reginald Howse, said: "There is nothing that even money can do for it."
> Take Kipling Block, built at the time of the British high noon in India. It was condemned for its inadequacy at the time the National Health Service started in 1948, and recommended for demolition. It was not demolished; today it houses 30 low-grade patients.
> Take the "Bear Pit", so called because it is like a zoo compound for polar bears. If you were to find children passing scraps of bread over the railings that surround it, you would not be surprised. Down below, the patients take occasional exercise. It is a forbidding place. So forbidding that the H.M.C. have had to use amenity fund money to provide a small, walled garden nearby.
> Brentry, one of Bristol's biggest mental sub-normality hospitals, with 420 patients, and 83 nurses - 12 below establishment - has for years been facing frustration. There is insufficient money to provide more than the bare essentials of life.
> Now that Mr Richard Crossman's Bristol visit has seemingly proved so abortive, the Hortham-Brentry H.M.C. are not very optimistic that life is going to be much easier in the forseeable future.
> What Brentry needs is not only more money for day to day expenses, and more

nurses and staff, but also capital for purpose built ward blocks. There is a more immediate need even than up-to-date dormitories. That is prefabricated workshops to get the frustrated patients out of gloomy wards. Between £15,000 and £20,000 - a mere bagatelle in the world of hospital finance - would enable the H.M.C. to provide them.

The gross annual revenue of the Hortham-Brentry group, which includes nine hospitals, is £940,000. This works out at 13 guineas a week per patient. What is needed to bring the figure up to 15 guineas a week, and make life just tolerable, is £1,050,000 a year. With that extra 42s. per patient, Brentry could be better staffed and buy better furnishings.

If Mr. Crossman's statement during his Stoke Park, Stapleton, visit, reflects the Government's present thinking on this type of hospital, the whole thing is just a pipe dream.

Even as things are at Brentry, the H.M.C. are currently overspending on revenue account by £22,000. This will be met by the additional £25,000 allocated as recently as September 30 by the Regional Hospital Board. This was originally intended to improve nursing standards and to give patients trifling extra amenities. All this is now out of the question. Mr Howse said: "You see how frustrating it is. We are always having to rob Peter to pay Paul."

There is, however a brighter side. Brentry has converted old tractor and farm sheds and pigsties at small cost into workshops to give patients occupational therapy. They have built a small swimming pool, a skittle alley; the League of Friends have given a club room. The pool was paid for from the profit made by the patients' club and the hospital staff social club. The cost of the alley was met by the H.M.C. income from a national hospital endowment fund.

Social Clubs, mothers' union branches, young wives leagues, and women's institutes are encouraged to pay organised visits to the hospitals in the group. Indeed several have visited Brentry during the past summer. "In this way," says Mr Howse, "the world outside our grey walls gets to know something about the life led by our mentally disordered patients. That part of it is encouraging."

But the overall problem of Brentry's backlog of vital work remains. New buildings involving the expenditure of a great deal of money. Who is to solve it? No one at Brentry really knows.[13]

The fears that Brentry would be passed over were not borne out as just prior to Mr Crossman's visit[14] the Government gave the Regional Hospital Boards a list of

'interim measures to improve hospital services for the mentally handicapped' and were asked to plan to achieve these within about five years, starting in 1970-1. ...

These interim measures included the improvement of patients' food (to which the top priority was to be given) and clothing; minimum space standards and maximum numbers of patients in any one ward to relieve the worst of the overcrowding; the provision of cupboards for all patients' personal possessions; specific staff-patient ratios for doctors, dentists and nurses and minimum numbers of domestic staff related to the size of the hospital and the degree of dependency of the patients; recruitment of staff for other forms of treatment; upgrading of buildings and furnishings; and adequate staff accommodation.

They also included the establishment of regular discussions between doctors, nurses and other therapeutic staff, staff training schemes, the encouragement of voluntary service and where appropriate the employment of a full-time organiser of voluntary services.[15]

As a result of this the RHB finally started to allocate money to the Mental Handicap Hospitals around Bristol. At Brentry the RHB authorised the building of two new prefabricated wards, Charlton and Blaise, and later two 'Coleshill' units (Leese and Anderson) so that the dreaded 'bear pit' of Kipling could be demolished and Baden Powell could stop being a dormitory.[16] Kipling was finally demolished in 1972[17] when Baden Powell was turned into a play therapy unit for the hospital. Haig and Allenby were emptied and then improved before reuse as wards.

As part of the new funding in 1970 it was decided to change the attire of the nurses from the uniform based on that of 1900 to one that would modernise the appearance of the hospital. The suits worn by the men was changed to a blazer and flannels and the women were placed in princess line dresses in various colours. However any change of uniform was not very obvious as the men continued to wear protective white jacket coats over their clothes. The committee resolved to look at alternatives to the white coats but do not seem to have implemented any changes.[18]

During this time the Government commissioned a new plan for the Mental Handicap services. In 1971 the new Government increased the spending plans to spend an extra £110 million on health and social services over the next 3 years and published a (then) revolutionary White Paper "Better Services for the Mentally Handicapped".[19] This White Paper solved the problem of the dilapidated old colonies by recommending the expansion of Community Care and the development by Social Services of 75 adult residential places per 100,000 population with the halving of hospital places to 55 per 100,000.[20] Similarly the local authorities should treble their day places to 150 per 100,000. They urged a radical reduction in the size of the new local authority hostels to be homes for a maximum size of 25. The paper still saw a strong role for hospitals and still considered that many people with a mental handicap needed hospital care but recommended that they now be housed in small units built on the sites of general hospitals, reflecting the need for medical care.

Prior to the publication of the White Paper, the Department of Health with Richard Crossman as minister, set out two principles of long term policy:[21]

a) that no new all-age hospitals would be built and that the local authorities would be responsible for the mentally handicapped except where hospitalisation is necessary on <u>medical</u> grounds (ie there should be no decanting to hospital on economic grounds alone); and

b) that hospitals should decant into the community as many mentally handicapped people as possible, and should provide hostels for those mentally handicapped people who do not in fact need full hospitalisation.

As part of the recommendations the government banned further building on the sites of old hospitals which held more than 500 inpatients.[22] This allowed development at Brentry but prevented it at both Hortham and Stoke Park who were desperate to further improve their slums as they saw little hope of a rapid discharge of inpatients to new community units. Everyone was pleased when the Hospital Advisory Service visited Bristol in 1971. As expected it recommended a large series of improvements that the RHB was under pressure to fund. Most spectacularly at Stoke Park the highly critical report was leaked to the press and a lot of correspondence was exchanged within the health service when Dr Heaton-Ward responded to the leak by telling the press that the report underestimated the problems and that some wards should be blown up![23] This resulted in the programme '24 Hours' showing a 19 minute film about Stoke Park on 2nd May 1972, which shocked the public and provoked a lot of further debate. It showed large numbers of highly dependant patients milling around with no daytime activity and being cared for by just one exhausted nurse, in scenes reminiscent of the novels of Dickens. The film was followed up by a series of articles in *The Listener* on the hospitals including a 4 page illustrated article on Stoke Park by Dr Heaton-Ward.[24] As a result of the publicity Stoke Park was provided with a series of 16 new wards over the next 12 years.

At Brentry, the 1971 Hospital Advisory Service report recommended a review of the management of the hospital group and the H.M.C. was forced to implement the Salmon nursing recommendations made in 1968. The HAS also recommended a simplification of administration so that the officers took over all day-to-day management from the committees, with the committees concentrating on matters of policy. Associated with this was an abolition of the hospital house committees who currently provided much of the day-to-day management. It criticised the Group Secretary Mr R W G Howse for not holding regular multidisciplinary meetings.[25] Howse recommended the abolition of the House Committees from the end of the year and the start of a new monthly multidisciplinary 'Officers Executive Committee' which would appoint the junior staff. In addition he created multidisciplinary teams to meet weekly or fortnightly in Brentry and Hortham. However these meetings were not very multidisciplinary as far as clinicians were concerned - only the head nurse and consultant psychiatrist sat on it alongside 5 support services managers, the group secretary and treasurer. Clinical multidisciplinary meetings had been happening at Hortham for several years by the time of the report and the nurses there had come to accept them. The HAS encouraged their introduction at Brentry despite the anxieties of the nurses who also had to cope with a change to their chain of authority with charge nurses reporting at times direct to the clinical team. In addition it was decided to implement the HAS recommendation to invite the chair of the Matron's committee to attend the H.M.C. alongside the Chair of the Medical Staff Committee, and to send copies of the H.M.C. minutes to the Head Nurses.[26] Though this change was small it represented a great symbolic change in the status of the nurse at the hospital. Nurses were now to be seen as being important in the running of the hospital and in the formulation of policy.

The Shakespeare Experiment

The 1970s saw a short but eventful experiment in therapeutic living at Brentry. In 1970 the young adult group on Shackleton was moved to Shakespeare ward in the lower village, and Shackleton used for the elderly.[27] This Shakespeare group was then the subject of a research project run by The Burden Institute with Dr Lower[28] and appears to have been run along more psychotherapeutic lines with the young males encouraged to take more responsibility. There were fewer nurses on the ward and there were periods of the day when no nurse was on the ward – ironically echoing the regime set up on Shackleton by Dr Rudolf in the 1930s. This regime was now a stress for the nurses, whose 'colleagues' at Farleigh were still being prosecuted for cruelty. They were no longer sure how they should react to the unruly patients. The project was likely to raise opposition. Soon after it started it was attacked for having only 7 of its 16 beds occupied and that

> Shakespeare patients appeared to be subject to a quite different code of discipline to that obtaining for other patients in the Hospital, and that the nursing staff in this Villa did not appear, under the terms of the research project to have adequate powers of discipline over these patients.[29]

As Dr Lower was away the concerns were noted and Brentry House Committee was asked to consider the Shakespeare Therapeutic Unit. They replied that:

> while they were of the opinion that this was a worthwhile unit, they had raised questions as to whether this type of unit was a matter for the Regional Hospital Board, rather than the Management Committee, whether it might be in a self-contained building in the community staffed by nurses other than those on a hospital establishment; and whether the unit should be allowed to continue with so many beds unoccupied in a hospital where other wards are very overcrowded.[30]

At the meeting, Dr Lower pointed out that the unit now contained 10 patients and another 4 were shortly to be admitted. He also pointed out that the camp which the patients from the unit had recently attended had proved very successful. The Hospital Management Committee decided to review the Unit at the next meeting when the report of the Hospital Advisory Service would be available. In fact the Hospital Advisory Service report did not refer to Shakespeare so the committee decided to make no further investigation 'for the time being' as the occupancy was higher.[31]

A year later in August 1972 it was noted that the ward fixtures were being severely damaged by the patients. When this was referred to the new Hospital Multidisciplinary Team[32] they recommended that the patients helped look after more of Shakespeare as they kept their day room in good order. This occurred and the damage seems to have lessened.

The lads who were admitted were a varied bunch. Dr Lower was prepared to accept for 'individual positive therapy' men who would otherwise have been sent to prison or Rampton. To many of the community workers and social workers around the south-west he was a hero. Several adolescents were admitted after stabbing close relatives, assault or theft. Others had been inpatients for some time, with recurrent acts of theft or temper outbursts. Some had sexually assaulted children or other residents. Some had been absconding to have dates with the local girls. Many had been repeatedly admitted and then discharged themselves. Some were of average (normal) intelligence.

Several continued to abscond when on Shakespeare, at least one stealing a car when out. There was often a problem with their food, when they ate all their allowances and begged supplies from the neighbouring wards.

A crisis occurred in November when the Hospital Management Committee was told that:

> Mrs S Price, Senior Psychologist was attacked by a male patient from Shakespeare Villa, threatened with a knife, subjected to indecent exposure of and possible rape by him, after she had taken the patient with two other male patients for an evening walk into Henbury as part of therapeutic treatment. …
> The Group Secretary referred to certain anxieties and reservations regarding the Shakespeare Ward expressed by the Management Committee … [in] 1971, and to the anxiety felt by the Chairman and himself regarding the position whereby in the course of their duties Mrs Price and other female staff, including domestic staff, could on occasions be alone with male patients, particularly the Shakespeare and similar patients, under circumstances involving risk to such staff, and stated that, at the request of the Chairman and as a matter of urgency he had issued to Dr Lower, the Responsible Medical Officer, and to Mrs Price a disclaimer on the part of the Management Committee of any liability or responsibility for the safety of Mrs Price or any other member of the female staff if they are alone with male patients from Shakespeare Villa; and furthermore he had issued an instruction that where patients were taken for walks or were brought back after they had absconded, a male nurse should be present. The Chairman and he also referred to the risks to the public and of adverse effects on the good name of the hospital, and on visitors and volunteers. Reference was also made by the Group Secretary and the Chief Male Nurse to incidents involving other patients and domestics on two occasions and the fact that patients subjected them to foul and abusive language. The Group Secretary warned the Committee of the possible accusation that they were taking inadequate precautions to protect staff and the public, and their liability in law if any other incident occurred.
> Dr Lower emphasised the essential need for an individual approach to the Shakespeare patients in their therapeutic treatment, and strongly deprecated any instruction which precluded female members of the therapeutic team from being alone with male patients on occasions; and he stressed that without this individual approach, the team's programme of treatment and rehabilitation would become impossible. In this connection, Mrs Price stated that she regarded incidents such as the one referred to as a normal hazard of her job.
> Resolved: (a) having regard to the remarks of Dr Lower as RMO for the Shakespeare Patients, to withdraw for the time being, and with reluctance and reservations, the disclaimer and instructions already issued by the Group Secretary regarding female staff being alone with male patients, but at the same time to confirm such action as having been right and proper at the time in the light of information then available. (b) To appoint a working party … to investigate in detail the position of female staff in relation to the treatment and rehabilitation of the Shakespeare and similar staff....[33]

The night female staff were withdrawn from the unit.[34] The full events of the assault were reported in the local press when it came to court:

> Richard Lee Belcher (23) indecently assaulted a senior woman psychologist in the hospital discotheque, Bristol Crown Court heard. Belcher admitted the offence.... It was said that he asked the woman to see the new discotheque lights. He exposed himself to her and brandished a knife. The Knife fell to the ground and she managed to kick it under the door. Belcher then placed his hands under her clothes. She managed to escape by saying she would go to the woods with him.
> It was said that Belcher had been sent to Brentry under a probation order. This followed a conviction for administering a noxious substance. He put weed-killer in his mother's tea. He was gaoled for six years.[35]

The nurses were, however now very worried about the unit, and seem to have lost any trust that they had in the project and Dr Lower. It upset the natural order of hospital discipline and made the nurses feel unsafe. This was not helped by six of the patients severely damaging and trying to drive off a nurse's car. As the nurse complained to the Head Nurse 'I am annoyed with the liberties being taken by these patients, which I am powerless to stop due to the therapeutic treatment they are receiving, but I am complaining about these patients interfering with my car.' The nervousness of the nurses about how to treat the patients was made worse by a series of articles on nursing. Journalists from the *Sunday People* obtained employment in several hospitals, including Hortham, and their experiences were published under the front-page headline "The bullies in our hospitals", condemning the rough handling of patients by nurses.[36] The nurses were now even more nervous of how to respond to the patients on Shakespeare. Matters came to a head in January 1974 when a male nurse was attacked. The unions forced the issue by going to the newspapers:

> Nursing Assistant Mr Hems was hit over the head repeatedly after intervening in a dispute between two male patients who were watching a football match on television.[37]
> It took place in Shakespeare ward late at night. Two male patients were fighting and Mr Hems stepped in to try to break it up. He was punched repeatedly in the face, receiving a black eye and severe bruising. ... He had to have stitches for facial injuries. He will be off duty for a week.[38]
> And staff at the hospital say the attack shows that Brentry patients are getting out of control. Discipline has disappeared since recent investigations into alleged cruelty towards mental patients, they said last night. Nursing assistants are taunted, sworn at and abused. ... [Mr Hems] told me last night that new methods of treatment in recent years meant that no discipline was given to patients in the ward where he was attacked.[39]

Mr Hems was so affected that in March he gave up his job as a nurse "because he felt he was a marked man".[40] His case was later mentioned in the Sunday Times when discussing violence to nurses.[41] Immediately after the attack the COHSE union representative 'requested' a meeting with the management board - a special meeting was arranged:

> Mr. Fullbrook, in thanking the Committee for arranging the meeting, stated that he had been requested by his members to bring forward certain points regarding the particular care and treatment of patients in Shakespeare Ward, as introduced by the responsible medical officer, and to voice, on behalf of nursing and other staff in relation to such care and treatment certain anxieties which had been highlighted by the incident referred to. He submitted the following points:
> (a) The majority of the patients on Shakespeare Ward were not classified as mentally subnormal and the nursing staff on the ward, who were trained and employed in the subnormality field, felt that it was not part of their contract to nurse those particular patients.
> (b) Nursing staff had no confidence in the treatment prescribed by the responsible medical officer on Shakespeare Ward; under such treatment patients evinced a bad attitude to work, a poor discipline, and a lack of respect

towards staff; patients were permitted to address all staff on the ward, including the responsible medical officer, by their christian names.

(c) Nursing staff had reported that Shakespeare patients leave the ward in the evening to visit local public houses returning to the ward at midnight with the explanation that they have only been for a walk; but no disciplinary action had been taken, with the result that such patients take advantage of the staff and undermine their confidence and authority.

(d) In regard to the incident of the attack by a patient, nursing staff had been astonished and appalled by attitude of the responsible medical officer who appeared to interpret as "mishandling" the action of the nursing officer concerned in attempting to separate two combating patients immediately prior to the attack.

(e) The nursing staff did not understand the particular therapy practised by the responsible medical officer on Shakespeare Ward, and they felt that the Shakespeare Unit should operate completely outside of the environment of a mentally subnormal hospital. The particular type of discipline, or lack of discipline, applying to the Shakespeare patients had inevitably spread to other patients in the hospital with adverse effects on those patients and on the work of nursing and other training staff generally. There had been bullying of older and weaker patients by the Shakespeare patients, accompanied in some instances with a demand for money or cigarettes.

(f) The psychologist on occasions issued instructions to nursing staff, some of whom, particularly the older officers, felt that instructions should come from the Consultants.

(g) There was generally a strong feeling amongst nursing staff in regard to Shakespeare Ward and the particular therapy practised there: certain staff were very reluctant to work there and, since the particular incident, female staff had been under strong pressure from their husbands not to work on that ward.

(h) Junior doctors sometimes countermand disciplinary measures taken by nurses, thereby undermining their authority.

(i) Nursing staff felt handicapped by a lack of disciplinary authority and would welcome guidance as to what authority they could exercise to correct patients.

In the ensuing discussion in the presence of the COHSE representatives the question was raised as to the application of multi-disciplinary management principles to the operation of the Shakespeare Unit but it did not appear that ward meetings in Shakespeare were run on MDM lines in the generally accepted sense of the term. Shakespeare Ward and the therapy practised there had not been the subject of discussion by the Hospital MDM Team although the team could discuss the problems with the trade union and report back to the Management Committee if the union wished.

With regard to the incident of the attack and the way in which assistance had been summoned by an older patient, it was accepted by the Committee that consideration should be given to the installation of an alarm system throughout the hospital which could be operated under similar circumstances in the future.

On being questioned as to any disciplinary powers of nursing staff, Mr. Fullbrook stated that such staff could not exercise such powers even to the limited extent of putting a patient to bed early or stopping his T.V. It was confirmed that the responsible medical officer could restrict or reduce cash issues of pocket money to patients and could delegate this power to nursing officers, but the balance of pocket money within the authorised allowance would still be credited to the patients' accounts; however, he could vary the allowance on therapeutic grounds.

Mr. Fullbrook and Mr. Smith then left the meeting and the Committee interviewed Mr. Garment, who reiterated a number of points previously raised by Mr. Fullbrook and suggested that more overtime should be available to nursing staff to overcome staff shortages.

The Committee RESOLVED (i) to express confidence in the nursing staff and sympathy with such staff in the problems and anxieties referred to: (ii) that, having regard to the effect which the operation of the Shakespeare Unit is having on other patients and staff throughout the hospital, to recommend to the

> Regional Hospital Board that the Unit be located outside the curtilage of the hospital: (iii) to request, through the Chairman of the Psychiatric Division, that the consultants should compile, for submission to the next meeting of the Committee, guidelines indicating disciplinary measures which could be exercised by nursing staff without reference to the consultants: (iv) to express concern to the Hospital MDM Team regarding the possibility of staff being unwilling to work on Shakespeare Ward, and the non-involvement of nursing staff in the MDM ward conferences for that ward.[42]

The Shakespeare research project closed within the month:

> Further consideration of Shakespeare - pointed out that it was no longer possible to obtain staff and that future staffing likely to be extremely difficult.
> With regard to guidelines on discipline - ...it was hoped to commence ... seminars in the course of the next 2-3 weeks. RESOLVED: a) to place on record the Committee's appreciation of the hard work and dedication to duty displayed by Dr Lower and the supporting staff in the running of Shakespeare. 2) Nevertheless to close the unit in its present form until such time as a complete establishment of suitably qualified and willing staff is available to man the unit. 3) The existing patients on Shakespeare be scattered into the general pattern of care by the RMO if necessary into wards under the care of another RMO. 4) In the meantime Shakespeare be reintegrated into the hospital (suggested transfer of female patients of Dr Bird's at Hortham). 4) express hope the seminars will commence within the next month.[43]

It is easy to see Shakespeare as a very unsuccessful experiment, but the clinical notes of the residents seem to indicate that many of them improved whilst on the ward. Most of them had a very disturbed background, and none were seen as easy to treat. It must be said that many of the older more able patients on the other wards had similar backgrounds and patients on the other wards, such as Darwin, were as troublesome and capable of such things as sexually assaulting or intimidating a junior male nurse.

The first Female Inpatients at Brentry

The Hospital Advisory Service report of 1971 recommended that Brentry start admitting female patients and children. It was decided not to admit children but to exchange an adult ward with Hortham and as a result Wellington was converted into the two wards of Westbury and Berkeley to receive women. One part of the conversion was to move the Billiard Table from the ward to the Play Therapy Building.[44] However the management committee were soon unhappy with the ward chosen by the medical staff for the exchange and by the use of seclusion:

> The Committee were informed that Wellington Ward had been modernised and divided into two wards for the reception of female patients, which had commenced on 1st November, 1973. [45]

The Chairman, Mrs Anderson then referred to a recent routine rota visit she had made to Brentry in the company of two other managers. They had paid a visit to Westbury Ward and were very distressed over an incident with a patient [XX] who was in the seclusion room and asked for their help. After this visit she had asked the Group Secretary to make further enquiries regarding her detention in the seclusion room and the history of any such detention whilst at Hortham prior to transfer. She had been surprised to learn that two months previously the patient had been in continuous seclusion at Hortham for almost three weeks.

She had also called for the seclusion book for Westbury Ward and noted that XX had been in the seclusion room for a week, and another patient had been in for over a week. Dr. Lower the responsible medical officer, was asked if he would give some information to the Committee regarding the two patients.

He felt that though she was attention seeking, he had been more successful in helping her with controlled management than anyone else had been up to the present. Her current appeal to the Mental Health Tribunal for discharge from detention had improved her behaviour but she still had recently absconded. Dr. Lower felt that she could be extremely dangerous but he did not want her to go to Rampton and that after 15 years of disturbed behaviour, she was being helped for the first time in her existence by some control.

With regard to the second patient, she had recently returned from Rampton and had become destructive. She would have to return to Rampton if she did not improve.

Dr.Lower answered numerous questions from members and explained that the initial reason for their detention in the seclusion room was that they were upsetting people generally, for example playing the record player at a high volume.

> With regard to the seclusion rooms, these are quite empty except that patients would have a strong mattress which could not be torn, strong bedding and a strong gown to wear. In seclusion when they had need to be apart from other people for some time, they did not have books or magazines very often as they could use these in a dangerous way. As far as bedding was concerned, this must be strong or it could be used for self-injury; if other articles were supplied, they could be used as instruments against staff when entering the room.
>
> The Chairman and members stated that they were under the impression that, following the Hospital Advisory Service report and the decision to bring female patients to Brentry, the type of patient would be such as would be suitable for social integration with the male patients and it would not be of the severely disturbed type now in Westbury Ward. The Chairman had also heard., whilst on a visit to Hortham, that it was intended to transfer physically handicapped female patients to Brentry and it transpired that these would be of a low mental grade similar to the patients in Dickens Ward.
>
> Members having asked all the questions they wished to put, Dr. Lower and Mr. Gilbert were asked to leave the room so that members could discuss the matter freely.
>
> The Group Secretary was asked if there had been any accidents to staff and he stated that two members of the staff had been bitten and a third kicked on the leg by [one patient who] had sustained bruises by bumping herself against the seclusion room door.... RESOLVED UNANIMOUSLY: (a) to strongly deprecate the introduction of patients into the new women's wards in view of the Committee's implied intention that the wards should be initially filled with suitable patients for social integration in accordance with their stated purpose for the improvement and development of the all male community at Brentry. (b) members were perturbed about the length of seclusion revealed, having particular regard to the lack of reasons given in the seclusion book. (c) that Staff should give in the book more lucid reasons or explanations for detention, the present system being grossly inadequate. (d) the reason for detention should be in the doctor's writing and not written in by the nurses. (e) that the Committee's resolutions in this matter should be drawn to the attention of the Board's Senior Administrative Medical Officer at they felt powerless to do anything further in that (i) the use of the seclusion rooms is a clinical matter: (ii) all consultants are employed by the RHB.[46]

The Management Committee were clearly unhappy with the medical management of the patients and were not happy when 'Patient XX' was discharged by Dr Lower shortly after the meeting and prior to the Mental Health Tribunal hearing.

> Dr G Russell as chairman of the Division, stated that neither he nor his consultant colleagues were in a position to comment on the use of security rooms within the context of the Special Units. He referred to a Joint report compiled in 1972 by the Royal College of Psychiatrists and the Royal College of Nurses, containing recommendations on the care and treatment of violent patients and the conduct of nursing staff in this context, and pointed out that this

report was still being considered by a Working Party appointed by the Department. ....
RESOLVED: to inform the acting Senior Acting Medical Officer of the RHB of the inability of the chairman of Division to comment on the use of security rooms. (b) to place on record and inform the RHB that the H.M.C. were not associated in any way with the discharge of the patient XX.[47]
Resolved to watch situation on Westbury and Berkeley.[48]

The straitjacket and seclusion or security room continued to be used on Westbury and less frequently, elsewhere on the site. It does though seem to have been used more with the women then the male patients. There were also seclusion rooms on Sick Ward (Colston) and Jellicoe and staff can recall both being in use at the same time. It has to be remembered that then, as now, it was often very difficult to get the police to remove a patient who was very violent or who physically threatened people. Staff were not given any formal training in how to restrain people effectively or safely, except that learnt from other staff 'on the job'. Seclusion was often resorted to as the only way of keeping people safe and this could last for a month or more if no-one agreed to remove the patient to another site. The final seclusion room was not closed until the 1980s.

Building and changes in activities

With the increased investment by the RHB the fabric and conditions at Brentry started to improve at last. One minor but significant improvement was that in 1971 the sewerage system was thoroughly cleaned to stop the toilet blocks from smelling so badly. In addition the Physiotherapist was given a work space and office, converted from the old disused mortuary. More lockers were provided for the patients as were some disposable toothbrushes.

The first new unit had been Charlton and Blaise, then a double ward Leese and Anderson were built in the lower village in 1972 and Kipling demolished. With the investment came an increase in recruitment and a reduction in overall bed numbers, as the Hospital Secretary was able to document in 1974:[49]

Year	No of pts	No of Ward Units	WTE Staff
1966	440	11	72
1971	420	12	106
1974	398	15	141 including 22 students and 5 cadets

However the reduction in beds was not totally welcomed as the salary of some officers was determined by the size of the hospital and a reduction below 400 affected some salaries.

The end of the farm at Brentry led to an application in 1972 for patients to be transported to work on the Purdown Farm and Horticultural training scheme. The transport cost for 10 patients was to be £2200 a year. The Committee were not prepared to pay this and suggested that the patients involved moved to Purdown.

> Secretary explained to the Committee that at Hortham and Brentry some years ago farm training schemes existed, there being cattle, pigs and poultry, in addition to large kitchen gardens. The farming side of the scheme was terminated because of the view of the Department that the scheme was being run at a substantial loss and the retention of farms could only be justified if essential to the therapeutic needs of the patients. Despite the fact that there was a larger number of higher grade patients at that time, the medical staff had been unable to supply patients in an adequate number to justify the retention of the farm and, in fact, 15 acres under cultivation also had to be given up as patients were not available even to keep the area tidy.[50]

At this time the relationship between the hospital secretary and the medical staff must have been strained given that the minutes appear to blame the medical staff for the lack of able patients at Brentry. The stresses of the Shakespeare experiment and of the seclusion of the Westbury patients must have exacerbated the strain.

Occupational Therapists were still not specifically employed and all therapy was done by nurses and trainers. Patients in the lower village would be taken to the industrial therapy unit, to fill moulds with concrete or assembling ballpoint pens. They attended the Play Therapy Unit at Baden Powell for painting, drawing, plasticine play and other similar activities.

The main force in the hospital at this time, though was always said to have been the Chief Male Nurse, Mr Gilbert. The place ran with military precision, with patients clean and ordered. He would visit wards without warning, often to try to catch out staff eating patient's food. As a result all wards had their lookouts, who would shout if anyone was coming. All patients stood up when he entered the room and you would have to have well polished shoes. One of the residents remembers having to make the beds with military precision – with the staff inspecting the accuracy of the hospital corners on the sheets.

The relationship with the public of Henbury and Brentry continued to have its ups and downs. Escapes still occurred but by the late 1960s most of those who wanted to leave had been discharged. The patients who wandered out of the grounds were still a source of concern for the community and the publicity around the Shakespeare experiment did not alleviate their concerns. Nor did such events as a brick being thrown over the boundary wall of the hospital by an unidentified patient and seriously damaging the radiator of a passing car.[51] The hospital, though was equally becoming suspicious of the community, particularly after the building of the Henbury council estate in the 1950s, which seemed to increase the number of people walking across the hospital lands. A footpath still ran across the grounds and along the woods and was a focus of this concern. In 1961 an attempt was made to close it as 'patients go on it and girls from the local housing estate walk on it with the patients nearby'.[52] This attempt failed and it was not until 7 years later[53] when the footpath on Knole Lane was improved that the committee succeeded in diverting the footpath after reaching a compromise with the Ramblers Association. The path was moved further away from the top recreation ground and at the same time the land on the far side of it was sold.[54] The eventual purchaser never appears to have erected the 'high unclimbable and suitable wall on the hospital side of the diversion' that was originally intended. The patients from Darwin and other more able wards continued to chat up the girls and boys who came onto the site and would often walk into the village with the girls.

When Leese and Anderson were built the contractors created a gate to Knole Lane to help their access to the site. It was decided to keep this access in favour of the pedestrian access at Park Field but later it was closed except for emergency vehicle access 'as if opened it would encourage children to use adjacent playing field, and patients to go onto the lane.'[55]

By 1972 the unwanted visitors had become a serious nuisance:

> It was pointed out that the pool had, over a considerable period, been subjected to acts of vandalism by trespassers, including the throwing in of broken bottles and the use of the pool as a toilet, and a letter which had recently been addressed to the Chief Constable, requesting all possible assistance in connection with such vandalism was read to the Committee.[56]

This approach to the police did not cure the problem though. The vandalism problem had increased over the decade and it was probably because of this that the local youth group was now refused the use of the Brentry playing fields. Due to the vandalism to the pool lining the sides of the pool were concreted in 1970 and the pool was covered in 1972 (Figure 9.1).

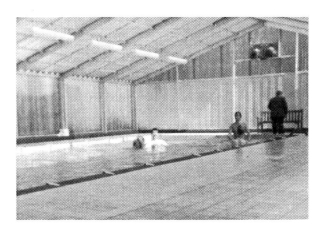

Figure 9.1: The Swimming pool in about 1973

There were other positives with the community though: Brentry League of Friends still held annual Gymkanas and fete days as it had during much of the 1960s and large numbers of volunteers were now being encouraged. This had started with the public relations officer, and increased by the voluntary services officer who was employed in the early 1970s. In February 1974 the Hospital Management Committee noted that under Mr Tom Malpas, the Voluntary Services Organiser for Brentry, over 1800 visitors from 35 Voluntary Services Organisations had visited the hospital and

> the committee were most impressed by the variety of ways and means in which these volunteers had been integrated into the functions of the hospital and the general care of patients. Particular projects referred to were the construction of an adventure playground, which would extend over a period of approximately two years, and the building of a sand yacht, in respect of which, the Weston-Super-Mare Sand Yacht Club were offering technical advice and instructions to patients. Reference was also made to a film which had been produced under the auspices of the Duke of Edinburgh's Award Scheme in which patients at Brentry, with the consent of relatives, would be appearing.
> It was mentioned that the Lions Club and Rotary Club were also taking an active interest in the welfare of patients at Brentry.
> It was agreed that suitable cinematograph equipment should be purchased which, amongst other functions, could be used to record progress on volunteer projects, particularly the adventure playground, and a vehicle for the use of the Organiser of volunteers for the transportation of patients and volunteers.[57]

Sports days continued, with staff crawling under the back of the beer tent to raid the drinks and others walking around with buckets of cigarettes for the patients. These days so not seem to have been attended by the public, except by invitation, and many of the rival participants came from other hospitals. Most came from Hortham but some came from Stoke Park, Purdown and Hanham Hall and some from Farleigh.

The 1972 Meeting

In 1972 Brentry celebrated its first 50 years of caring for adults with mental handicap. Few major celebrations seemed to have occurred at the hospital, and the anniversary seems to have passed the patients by. However on the 13 April 1972 the South West division of the Royal Medical Psychiatric Association (later to become the Royal College of Psychiatrists) held its meeting at Brentry. They received talks based on the work going on at Brentry: Dr Lower spoke on 'Individual Positive Therapy and change of personality' and Ms Price, the Senior Clinical Psychologist talked on 'Involvement, dependency and realistic fantasy – problems of assessment'. After a sherry reception and five course lunch, the meeting was addressed by Dr Jancar on the history of Brentry.[58]

Notes

[1] Personal recollection of Dr John Harrison.

[2] *Report of the Committee of Inquiry into Allegations of Ill-Treatment of Patients and other irregularities at the Ely Hospital, Cardiff.* [Cmnd.3975] London: H.M.S.O., March 1969.

[3] *Report....* Para 488.

[4] *The Times* 12 Aug 1969: 2a-c

[5] *The Times* 13 Aug 1969: 2g-h

[6] W.Alan Heaton-Ward: 'Perspective'. *Bulletin of the Royal College of Psychiatrists.*(1989) **13**: 225-30 (page 229).

[7] H.M.C. 9 Jan 1969 Special Meeting

[8] Hortham/Brentry Committee 26 March 1970 Minute 65(51)

[9] H.M.C. 26 November 1970 Minute 38/29

[10] H.M.C. 26 November 1971 Minute 52

[11] H.M.C. 1 June 1973 Minute 21

[12] *Daily Mirror* 5 December 1973

[13] *Bristol Evening Post* 5 November 1969

[14] Promise of Cash for Mental Hospitals. *The Times,* 8th October 1969: 3a

[15] Department of Health and Social Security: *Better Services for the Mentally Handicapped.* [Cmnd.4683] London: H.M.S.O., 1971. Paras 226-8.

[16] H.M.C. Minutes 30 July 1970 Minute 21.

[17] H.M.C. Finance Committee minutes 28 June 1972 minute 27 and 24 October 1973 Minute 59. Demolition cost £715 and £645 to remove the rubble and re-level the area

[18] H.M.C. Minutes 30 July 1970 minute 7.

[19] Department of Health and Social Security: *Better Services for the Mentally Handicapped.* [Cmnd.4683] London: H.M.S.O., 1971.

[20] *Better Services* ... Table 5.

[21] Charles Webster *The Health Services since the War, Volume 2: Government and Health Care, the National Health Service 1958 – 1979.* London: The Stationery Office, 1996, page 240-1.

[22] *Better services...* para 242.

[23] W.Alan Heaton-Ward: 'Perspective'. *Bulletin of the Royal College of Psychiatrists.*(1989) **13**: 225-30 (page 229).

[24] *The Listener* 8 June 1972 **87**: 745-8.

[25] H.M.C. minutes - report of Multidisciplinary meeting held 23 September 1971

[26] H.M.C. 21 October 1971 Minute 44

[27] H.M.C. 28 October 1970 Minute 2.

[28] MHC 26 November 1970 Minute 40

[29] H.M.C. 27 May 1971, minute 8

[30] H.M.C. 29 July 1971 Minute 19/8.

[31] H.M.C. 30 September 1971 Minute 34/19

[32] H.M.C. 4 August 1972 Minute 32.

[33] H.M.C. 1 December 1972 Minute 49.

[34] H.M.C. Minutes 2 February 1972. Minute 57/49

[35] Evening Post 24 Jan 1973.

[36] *Sunday People* 7 January 1973

[37] Evening Post 10 Jan 1974.

[38] Evening Post (second edition) 7 January 1974 with a photo of Mr Hems' injured face

[39] *Western Daily Press* 7 Jan 1974 with a photo of Mr Hems' injured face

[40] *Evening Post* March 11 1974, page 2ab. Also reported in *Western Daily Press* 15 Jan 1974.

[41] *Sunday Times* 24 Feb. 1974 page 5a this says he was off work for 3 weeks.

[42] H.M.C. minutes of special meeting 14 January 1974.

[43] MHC Minutes 14 February 1974 Minute 57/54

[44] H.M.C. Finance Committee Minutes 17 February 1971 Minute 126.

[45] H.M.C. 7 December 1973 Minute 54

[46] H.M.C. 7 December 1973 Minute 54

[47] H.M.C. 14 Feb 1974

[48] H.M.C. 1 March 1974

[49] H.M.C. minutes of special meeting 14 January 1974.

[50] H.M.C. Finance Committee 26 September 1973 Minute 49

[51] Hortham/Brentry Committee - Finance Committee 18 April 1961 Minute 6.

[52] Hortham/Brentry Committee 25 Jul 1961 Minute 22.

[53] H.M.C. 31 Jan 1967 Min 53

[54] Hortham/Brentry Committee 28 May 1968 minute 8; 26 November 1968 minute 37/30.

[55] Hortham/Brentry Building works committee 11 July 1973

[56] H.M.C. Finance Committee 26 July 1972 Minute 40.

[57] H.M.C. 1 March 1974 Minute 68

[58] Minutes and programme for the meeting are in the Royal College of Psychiatrists archives. Dr Jancar published his talk: J. Jancar: Fifty years of Brentry Hospital (1922 - 1972). *Bristol Medico-Chirurgical Journal* 1972 **87**:23.

Southmead Health Authority

The NHS was reformed in 1974.[1] The H.M.C.s were replaced by Area Health Authorities that operated District Management Teams. The Hortham-Brentry Hospital Management Committee was abolished and the operation of all the units managed by the Hortham-Brentry H.M.C., apart from St Mary's, Painswick, were transferred to the Southmead District Management Team under the Avon Area Health Authority (Teaching).

For the first time in its existence, Brentry now became part of a group of acute and general hospitals with a totally different ethos to that of the mental subnormality services. Much of its administration was dispersed amongst the District Management Team. It was now being managed by people who could compare the quality of care with that of the acute sector and enabled easy access to the specialist staff of Southmead such as Dietitians and Speech and Language Therapists. On the negative side its funds were now liable to being quietly diverted to bail out overspending in the local acute sector, and at times there does not seem to have been one manager who was clearly identifiable as the person responsible for the hospital.

This decade also marks the start of the move of the attention of heath staff caring for people with a mental handicap from the colony-hospital to working in the community. This would generate a new pattern of care, a new language and a lot of anxiety as well as hope.

Medical and nursing staff changes

In the 1970s Brentry was a stronghold of the COHSE union with 300 members in 1974.[2] As a result the hospital was involved in all the national COHSE disputes on pay. One major dispute was a pay claim in May – July 1974, when in May the COHSE staff walked out for two hours and then started a ban on overtime working and a ban on working with agency nurses. Most of the Bristol hospitals were severely affected until it was resolved. Again in June 1982 national industrial action was threatened when two staff at Brentry, Mr Patrick McManus and Mrs Mary Parry faced disciplinary measures for not revealing the names of staff who stopped work for an hour during a TUC day of action.[3]

Despite all these disputes the life of the patients did not dramatically improve. In 1975 the Avon Area Health Authority had to direct the Southmead Health Authority to reduce the numbers on Haig and Allenby from 66 to 48 due to the complaints of overcrowding. At the time it was stated that these were felt to be two of the worst wards in the area.[4] The District Management Team [D.M.T.] agreed to prioritise this over demands to replace wards at Southmead. A year later the hospital secretary still felt compelled to write to the *Bristol Evening Post* saying that that the day cover on wards at Brentry was worse than ten years previously although there were now 80 fewer patients.[5]

The D.M.T. noted that Brentry had many problems. The resident population was ageing and the wards were becoming unsuitable with their staircases. The Crossman prefabricated units of Blaise, Charlton, Leese and Anderson were already a maintenance liability and needed replacing 'within 10 years'.[6] This was also the year of national financial crisis and in June the Department of Health announced that it would sell off surplus hospital land. As a result a final 18.5 acres at Brentry was sold to the Bristol Corporation at a price of £434,000. After this Charlton and Blaise had major repairs in 1979[7] and these 'temporary' wards remained in use until 2000, the year Brentry closed. The ward upgrades unfortunately led to the loss of the offices for the psychologists at Brentry and they were forced to move to share the offices of their colleagues in Hortham, with four of them crammed into two small offices, much to their annoyance. This did not help their relationships with the medical staff who kept their more spacious offices at Brentry.

However the D.M.T. was now preoccupied with the old care homes in Bath that had been inherited with Hortham and Brentry. It was difficult to manage the homes in Bath, when the focus of the team was the west side of Bristol. In August 1976 the District Administrator suggested reusing Berwick Lodge as a children's unit, closing the children's unit at Rockhall in Bath. This did not occur and it was then suggested that Rockhall was moved to accommodation at Brentry, which also did not occur.[8] Rockhall closed by moving children to Hortham and then Rockhall was used for a short time as a holiday home for Brentry and Hortham.

The Divisional Nursing Officer then proposed that Berwick Lodge change to elderly women, noting that for the last few years the unit had been used as an extension of Brentry, housing 31 low dependency men, few of whom could find work in this rural setting so far from Bristol. He said that being an extension of Brentry failed to give it an identity - it had never developed any character and had remained institutional and impersonal (it 'has remained a high grade doss house' according to Mental Health Guardians). He noted that when the men were transferred to St Brenda's Hospital whilst the Lodge was repaired they had benefited. It was proposed that half the men disperse through the current Hostels in Bristol and be replaced by elderly women 'who could not benefit from living in Bristol'. The Community Health Council strongly resisted this plan for the ladies and nothing happened. The future of Berwick Lodge was finally settled when it was badly damaged by a fire in 1979. It was closed and sold to the Freeways Residential Trust on 27 March 1981.

At this time the opening of St Michael's Maternity Hospital in 1975 gave the D.M.T. an opportunity. The services at Mortimer House maternity unit had moved to Southmead and it could be closed as could two other maternity units – the 12 bedded Knoll at Clevedon was proving expensive as was the Thornbury maternity unit which was rarely reaching 60% occupancy.[9] After two years of planning, Ladymead House and Miles House were closed and the elderly ladies living there moved to Mortimer House in Clifton on the 3rd May 1977.[10] At the same time four ladies were moved from Downleaze Nursing home, where the Hortham-Brentry H.M.C. had contracted four beds (and where technically they were still inpatients), presumably to relieve some of the overcrowding in previous years.[11]

The White Paper of 1971 recommended that Local Authorities developed local hostels. Little of this happened in Avon but in 1978 an Area Health Authority advisor suggested that the hostels managed by the D.M.T. were transferred to Social Services. This sent a shock wave through the nursing staff who managed the hostels. There was a flood of letters of protest from the matrons of each hostel, from the psychology team and the medical staff. They all complained that the move would compromise nurse training and lower the moral of the nursing staff. They complained that the transfer would enable the local Social Services to avoid their duty to create more hostels. The Area Health Authority buckled and agreed that it was a 'premature proposal'.[12] The hostels were eventually transferred to Southmead Community Care Trust in 1989.

The morale of the nurses was not improved by the governmental committee of enquiry into Mental Handicap Nursing. The Jay Committee published its report in 1979 and made some wide reaching proposals that have been echoed in all later reports:

> 89. As a Committee we have identified three broad sets of principles which in combination underpin our thinking:[13]
> a) *Mentally handicapped people have a right to enjoy normal patterns of life within the community.*
> b) *Mentally handicapped people have a right to be treated as individuals.*
> c) *Mentally handicapped people will require additional help from the communities in which they live and from professional services if they are to develop to their maximum potential as individuals.*
> 91. c) *Any accommodation provided for adults or children should allow the individual to live as a member of a small group.*
> 93.a) *Mentally handicapped people should use normal services wherever possible.*
> c) *'Specialised' services or organisations for mentally handicapped people should be provided only to the extent that they demonstrably meet or are likely to meet additional needs that cannot be met by the general services.*

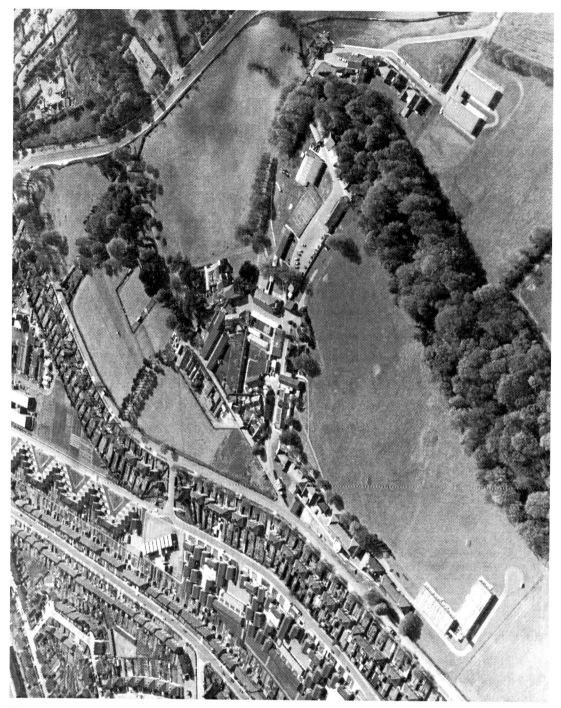

Figure 10.1: Ariel view of Brentry Hospital in 1975

The report noted that the student intake for mental handicap nursing had been falling and recommended a new training for staff, common to health service staff and local authority staff: the Mental Handicap Residential Care Worker.

The report was focussing on the long-term residential care needs of people and did not consider the role of community nurses or of nurses in assessment and treatment units. The specialist Community Mental Handicap Nurse was being advocated by the National Development Team. However the Jay report failed to see a future for mental handicap nurses in residential care and thereby made them feel even more insecure and unsure about their own future.

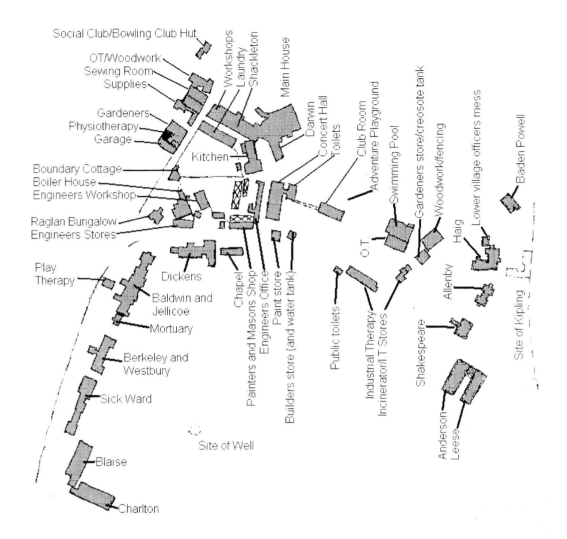

Figure 10.1 (cont): Explanation of image.

Another change had happened for the social workers who worked in the hospital. Prior to 1974 they had been employed by the health service and had an important role in the followup of people who were about to move out of hospital. Now they became part of the work-force of Social Services, which caused a lot of tensions as they changed their work practices to fit those of social services.

Dr Harrison came to work as a General Practitioner/ Clinical Assistant at Brentry in 1977, when it started a contract with his group practice to act as the GP's for the inpatients. He remembers it well.

> When I nervously attended my interview with Dr Lower, I found that the interview lasted a bare four minutes. It was enough that I had been trained at the same London Hospital as he, and that was it. I gained the impression of a quiet, controlled, rather distinguished gentleman of the old school. I crept thankfully away, to be intercepted just short of the gate by a harassed nurse to be told to see Mr Ryan Sir at once! I found a grizzled sharp-eyed Irishman wearing a military style uniform buttoned to the neck in the style of Army Blues, which his deputy also wore. This interview was the kind I had been dreading – an intensive review of my birth, breeding, education and experience for some 50 minutes. He, clearly, was not going to allow anyone he disapproved of working in HIS hospital. An amazing man. Fortunately I passed.

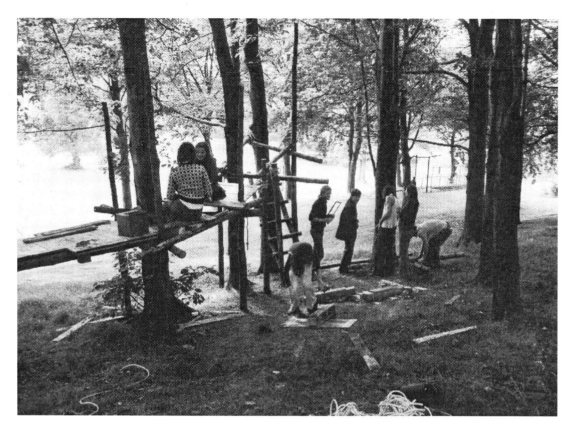

Figure 10.2: Building the adventure playground – in the background is the road to lower village.

> I found Brentry to be a quiet, orderly world where all nursing matters were efficiently organised, as were the patients. This was entirely due to the man at the top, Mr Ryan Sir. He was always called that.
> Because epilepsy was poorly controlled in these days much of my time was spent treating severe fits, or diagnosing fractures and carpet burns or sewing up gashes sustained in the fit.[14]

Ironically Mr Ryan was not the chief male nurse, but a charge nurse. Dr Harrison found that things were arranged differently to Hortham. At Hortham all physically ill patients were transferred to the Sick Ward, which operated as a miniature hospital. Brentry had a Sick Ward for the seriously ill but most of the ill patients were cared for on the wards. The nurses wanted to care for the patients through their illnesses. The Sick Ward did not function as a physical nursing ward – few of the nurses had a general nursing training, and there was little special equipment on it. The result was that the Clinical Assistants visited most wards each time they visited, rather than just the sick ward as at Hortham.

Patients and Activities

For all the changes and overcrowding 1975 saw the completion of an adventure playground and play area, built by voluntary workers from Henbury Comprehensive over two years with the encouragement of the voluntary services manager and money from the hospital (Figure 10.2 and 10.3). The intention was for a two acre adventure playground. What was built included some high towers and walkways that were not appreciated by the nursing staff: one recalls one of the residents who had epilepsy climbing to the top of the tower and refusing to come down. The ward staff ended up standing around wondering how they could get him down safely or if they waited what was the chance he would have an epileptic fit and fall off?

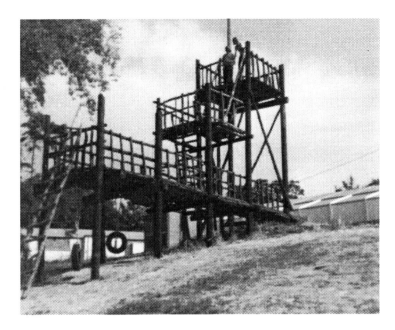

Figure 10.3: The tower in the Adventure Playground. Swimming pool is on right.

In addition it was soon found to be a honey-pot for the adolescents of the neighbourhood, who themselves were an attraction for the 'naughty boys' of Brentry and the delinquent lads of the neighbourhood. The adventure playground appears to have been quietly demolished within a couple of years.

With the loss of the fields and farming, the main day-time activity of the inpatients was in Industrial Therapy and Occupational Therapy. An occupational therapist, Gina McKellar, was the first person employed, and came to manage the Industrial Therapy as well as the Occupational Therapy department. Industrial Therapy still comprised such activities as assembling ball point pens and making concrete slabs and was generally repetitive and boring work. The 'old pen shop' was converted from the old agricultural buildings, namely the piggery. By 1980 they were no longer assembling pens but were sorting out bottle tops and assembling pots for bubble blowing. In the 1970s a 'New Pen Shop' was built next to the swimming pool and when the pool was covered over the buildings appeared as one. By 1980 this was being used for Occupational Therapy, making rugs and stools and other similar craft work. Next to this building was the woodwork room, where concreting was no longer done, but they assembled fencing and made bundles of wood for fire-lighting. This room had a large vat of creosote for dipping the fences in.

The swimming pool continued in use, as did the tennis court next to it and the social club, but during the 1970s the cost of running the pool led to it being closed, despite an active campaign to keep it open. In the 1980s there was an active attempt to recondition the pool so it could be reopened but the task was unsuccessful due to continued vandalism. The changing rooms were used by the sports groups until the pool building and new pen shop were burnt down in a series of fires that occurred around Brentry in about 1983 and included a fire in Jellicoe. A temporary member of staff was suspected but nothing was proved. The pool was then filled in and an era of swimming ended.

With the burning down of the new pen shop, or OT department, it moved into Baden Powell where it stayed for many years. One member of the OT staff also worked in the undercroft of Haig with 6 of the residents from Haig. This room was used by the barber every Thursday afternoon. The patients had to queue for the afternoon as they were processed in order, often 'borrowing' equipment from the room whilst they waited. The nurses would rediscover the equipment over the next week.

There were two other day care areas – the Play Therapy building was behind Jellicoe and was operated by nurses for the more handicapped patients. There was a more specialised woodwork shop opposite the sewing rooms, by the staff social club, which made garden furniture and did burnt poker work.

The Occupational Therapists became quite active in helping residents develop the skills for living in the community. In the mid 1980s an Occupational Therapist and Nurse were employed to assess patients for resettlement. They started in Boundary Cottage as a training house as the engineer had moved out some time previously. Patients would live at the cottage for two weeks, during the day. The cottage quickly proved uninhabitable and the resettlement assessment project moved to Raglan bungalow.

The patients still tended to all go on holiday in batches, with a summer camp booked for a season by the D.M.T., at such places as Boverton. In 1976 there was a serious plan to buy a holiday camp as a permanent holiday site for the patients. A coal board 'holiday camp' in Llanwit Major was due to be purchased with the support of the A.H.A. but the wooden huts were felt to be too dilapidated and the facilities of the camp too poor to merit purchasing.[15] The dilapidation was severe – the groups that visited had a problem finding habitable huts and the swimming pool was a ruin. It was decided to use the Knoll in Clevedon as a holiday home. Rockhall was also used for a few years after the children moved out in 1981 to Hillside, but the offer of the Stoke Park 'holiday' premises in Albert Road, Clevedon were rejected.

The growth of psychologists and multidisciplinary team working meant that several nursing practices were tighter regulated such as the procedure of 'Time Out' as a 'training activity' (in theory preventing the encouragement of behaviour by removing any reward from occurring after it). The problem with Time Out is that it can easily in practice become one of seclusion and punishment. A new procedure was drawn up by the psychologists and approved by all in 1978. It stressed that any Time Out procedures must be discussed with medical, psychological and nursing staff and *written down*.[16] Nursing staff were not to carry out Time Out of their own devising.

A new consultant psychiatrist arrived in 1979 and with it the wards were re-divided between the medical staff so each had a cross section of the patients in Brentry. The new consultant Dr Ockelford was to be responsible for Anderson, Baldwin, Blaise, Haig, Shackleton and Westbury. Dr Lower was now responsible for Charlton, Darwin, Dickens, Jellicoe, Leese, Shakespeare and Berkeley. Dr Gordon Russell would keep an interest by looking after Allenby.[17] There were clinical assistants and medical trainees on the wards as well. One recalls life at Brentry as being grim. The nurses would not allow her to visit the lower village at night and always brought to the top village any patient who needed a nocturnal medical review.

Brentry and the Community

The slow opening up of the Brentry site had an unwelcome effect that became prominent in the 1970s. The neighbouring youths started to come onto the Brentry site, walking their dogs or using the adventure playground, but also breaking into and stealing from wards and threatening or mugging staff and residents alike. This first hit the newspapers in 1975 when a nursing assistant was attacked.

> Youths with air rifles are terrorising mentally handicapped patients in Bristol's Brentry hospital ...The attackers, believed to be teenagers, have shot out several windows of the hospital.... And on Friday a gang of teenagers attacked nursing assistant Mr Robert Simmons, aged 21, in daylight, leaving him with bruises and head injuries. .... "We report each incident to the police but by the time a patrol car arrives the boys have fled"...Mr Simmons said ... a gang of teenagers had been roaming the grounds. "I was just going out for a paper when they threw me to the ground and kicked me round the head and arms. It

was very frightening. ... I know they have shot conkers at patients with catapults, hitting two of them in the head and neck. And female nurses have had insults hurled at them by the same boys." [18]

Security guards were employed but troubles continued and at times were blamed onto the security staff themselves.

Controversy and rumour again swept Brentry in August 1976 when a Night Sister, Mrs Susan Donaghue was murdered at her flat in Downleaze.[19] Her battered body was found by her boyfriend, a carpenter at Brentry, Dennis Foote, on Thursday 5th August when he went round to find out why she had not turned up for work. She had phoned in sick the previous day and a friend had stayed with her that evening. It was thought that she had been killed in her bedroom between 12.15am (when the friend left) and 7.30am (when Mr Foote found her), battered over the head with an old police truncheon she kept by her bed. Mrs Donaghue had worked at Brentry for only 3 years as a night nurse and lived alone in a bed-sit with few visitors, though she was a well-liked nurse. Because of her isolation the police could not tell if anything had been stolen. There were rumours of thefts and rape but the police did not confirm this. At the scene was the old truncheon, marked BD19 and thereby identified as coming from the Port of Bristol Docks Police before 1947. Also in the room was an old pair of size 6 men's pigskin driving gloves covered in blood. The police immediately tried to interview all the staff and patients at Brentry. They extensively interviewed and searched one patient and his ward before going on to interview over 5000 people but a month later they had to admit that they were no closer to finding her murderer. To this date no one has been charged with her murder but rumours still abound.

As well as the community coming to Brentry with volunteers working with the residents and manning the League of Friend's shop, Brentry staff also now went out into the Community. One of the first had been Dr Jancar who in the 1960s had started outpatient clinics at the Bush Training Centre in south Bristol. In 1975 Barbara Castle set up the National Development Team [NDT] to advise the Department of Social Services and Health on strategy and how to implement the 1971 White Paper. The NDT published a series of very influential pamphlets from 1976 on community services. In 1977 it advocated the setting up of Community Mental Handicap Teams as specialist teams to help children in the community.[20] It also recommended short-term residential facilities.[21] For hospitals it commented on the lack of use of hearing aids and spectacles due to the attitudes of staff and advocated personalised clothing, footwear and personal possessions. It celebrated the increased availability of pocket money for hospital residents.[22] It advocated joint community registers held by Social Services and Health to help planning and this was agreed locally in 1977.[23]

The NDT recommended the creation of Community Units[24] as a solution for areas where there was no hospital provision for the mentally handicapped. These were to be hospitals in the community, of 10 to 24 places and used in part to house residents nearer their families and in part for short-term stays. The Brentry Hospital Administrator, Mr Sykes, suggested that the Lower Village be turned into such a unit.[25] He suggested that after alterations, the empty Baden Powell and also Shakespeare be used by the Community Team as a Community Hospital. He pointed out that for the first 5 years the Team would only be able to use Baden Powell, Shakespeare and a third ward, whilst seventy long stay residents would remain in the village. It was to be hoped that the whole of the lower village would become a community hospital, but this was not to be expected until 'the 1990s'. In the meantime it was felt that this community unit would meet the suggestions of the NDT by being autonomous though it was an integral part of the hospital. This was discussed for the next year but not implemented. The NDT's proposal was for community hospitals where no other services existed, such as would have happened if the Knoll in Clevedon had been turned into one. They were not proposing turning parts of old hospitals into these units. However Baden Powell was renovated and adapted, including installing a two-way mirror, prior to the project being abandoned and Occupational Therapy taking over the building.

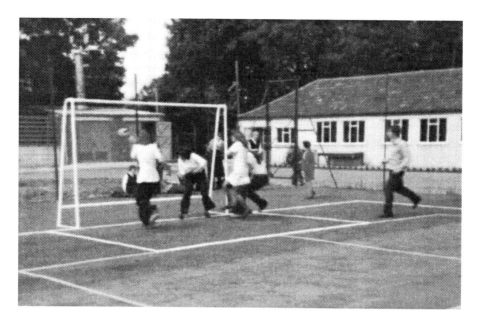

Figure 10.4: Playing football in about 1975 – the old piggery/ I.T. shed is on the right.

With the arrival of Dr Sylvia Lewis (later Carpenter) in 1983 there was a drive to create a Community Mental Handicap Team. A nurse was employed and based in Baden Powell with the community OT. The Community Mental Handicap Team for the area around Brentry was never to have a home for the whole team until 26 years later when the Health Service members of the Adult team at last moved in together, without social services. Ironically the base they eventually found was Baden Powell, at a time that the Lower village was again being suggested as a small Community Hospital for people with a Learning Disability.

One minor symbolic change at about this time was the demolition of the Gate Lodge, built in 1825 at the entrance to the 'private drive' to the main house. It was normally occupied by the deputy chief nurse and the last occupant was Jo Carpenan. The 1975 aerial photograph appears to still show it (Figure 10.1). There is now little trace of either the lodge garden or the building. The white wooden gate now stood alone, until it was too rotten to open and the driveway was closed to traffic in the later 1990s. Another change was the destruction of the conservatory attached to the house by a falling tree in a storm in about 1980.

Mental Health Act 1983

The 1980s saw a new Mental Health Act, to replace the 1959 act. It changed the term of Subnormality to Mental Impairment and allowed for the long term detention of psychopaths and people with mild mental impairment without the need of a criminal charge. The effect of the Act at Brentry was fairly minor, especially when compared with the changes enforced by the 1959 Act.

Southmead District Health Authority

In 1982 Southmead Health Authority became Southmead District Health Authority with the abolition of Avon Area Health Authority. A few years later Alan Carpenter replaced Rosemary Grant as the unit manager for the Mental Handicap Unit, managing Hortham and Brentry, along with The Knoll, Mortimer House, Berwick Unit (the old maternity unit in Thornbury), Chasefield and Hillside Houses.

At this time Brentry did not have a high reputation. Despite its 35 year association with Hortham it was seen by many from outside as having changed little and being full of archaic practice. It was also seen as being difficult to change due to the strong and militant union presence. It still operated long shifts, with two charge nurses of equal rank managing opposite teams on a ward. Student nurses at the time recall the way they would be left alone on the ward whilst some charge nurses had 'meetings' on other wards. Several have recalled drinking in the social club in the evening with staff who had left the ward they were in charge of to come drinking and were encouraged to stay by other staff there. Several staff recall the Regional Nurse Advisor being ordered off a ward by its drunk charge nurse after she commented that the ward looked rather institutional. The charge nurse is said to have gained local kudos from the nurses because of this. This attitude changed slowly over the 1980s as some staff left, some died and some were demoted in reorganisations or disciplined for offences. The staff social club closed amid some scandal and a staff suicide, and staff had to sometimes use the patients' social club. The real major change eventually came at the end of the 1980s when a lot of residents and staff from Hortham came to Brentry. However Brentry was not seen as the worst of the hospitals in Bristol. There were many very good staff and Brentry was in the forefront in some areas. For example it was the first of the two sites to employ female staff to work with male patients and it was Brentry who first employed Occupational Therapists.

One big change that hit Brentry was that crown immunity was removed from all hospital sites. Up to now the presence of crown immunity enabled the hospital to keep areas unchanged that were so dangerous or unhealthy that they would ordinarily have led to prosecution. Now health and safety concerns had a legal bite and the pressure was on to bring the wards up to a reasonable standard.

Closure Plans

During the 1980s Southmead planned the closure of the old hospitals of Brentry and Hortham. In 1975 the long term plan of the Regional Health Authority was that Brentry was closed and Hortham reduced to 179 adult beds and 43 childrens beds.[26] However economics and other realities had changed this plan. Though Hortham was seen as the more progressive hospital, it was the more isolated and thought to be a more valuable site being close to the motorway. It was decided to close Hortham first, moving the majority of people into small residential care homes.

The plan announced in October 1984 was for the closure of Hortham and the run down of Brentry over ten years with a community hospital developed on the Brentry site.[27] However the plans did not go down well at Brentry. Mr Alan Williams and Mr Les Fulbrook, charge nurses and COHSE officials reported to the press that 'some patients are in a state of panic and are reduced to offering cash to nurses in a last-ditch bid to stay in Brentry.' COHSE 'slammed the entire resettlement scheme as ill-conceived and rashly put together.'[28] The nurses later accused management of harassing them and discussed action with their national officers – 'we were summoned by management who demanded an explanation and wanted to know what patients and staff we had referred to'. The manager, Mr Alan Carpenter, said in response 'we were concerned that some of our residents might have some anxieties about the future of Brentry. We spoke to Mr Fulbrook to try and get some better idea of who they might be so that we could allay those fears. He was unable to help us.'[29]

The strategic plan that existed in 1985,[30] noted that it started at the 1984/5 bed allocation of 241 inpatients at Brentry and 395 at Hortham. The South Western Regional Health Authority policy was that the district of origin was responsible for resettling patients from the old hospitals. However for Brentry this was little use as many came from out of region, and their districts of origin would not be bound by the South Western rules. In the Southmead Mental Handicap Hospitals and Hostels there were 332 people from Southmead, Frenchay and Bristol and Weston Authorities, 53 from Gloucester and Cheltenham, 59 from Bath, 34 from elsewhere in the Region, 84 from the Wessex region other than Bath and 178 from other Regions. Gloucester had so many due to the 1920s commitment of Gloucestershire to the enlargement of Brentry Colony. The Plan was to run down Brentry at a rate of 20 - 40 patients a year from 1987 to 1994 when it would stay at 44 beds, and Hortham would be closed by 1991. Only small units would be used for resettling its residents. However the plans were reduced in about 1989 when Bath Health Authority who was in Wessex Region, announced that it did not have the money or obligation to repatriate the 60 patients from Bath that lived in Brentry and Hortham. Soon after this the whole resettlement project had to be rethought when it became clear that Southmead Health Authority had no additional money to put into resettlement but also needed to close Hortham Hospital on schedule to release money to enable other developments in the acute sector.

In the middle of all of this, in October 1988 Dr Fairburn died unexpectedly and suddenly. It came as an additional and symbolic blow to the hospitals as he was well liked and respected as the senior consultant, though his recent work load in Bath had prevented him from having much input into the hospitals. As a tribute the new respite care home in Little Stoke was named after him.

Hortham had to be closed in December 1991 by abandoning the avowed principle of using small homes and by using several large nursing homes. During this time few people were resettled from Brentry. Brentry was not run down but was topped up with staff and older residents from Hortham. Three houses for a total of 15 people were built on the edge of Brentry, in Robin Close, and opened in April 1992 to house those people from Hortham who were felt to be not able to be discharged, even after Brentry closed. Other groups were moved over as groups. Haig was used to house the men from Hortham's James Ward. Darwin was renamed Shannon and a small secure fenced compound attached to it to accommodate the residents of Hortham's Failand ward. Charlton ward was renamed Willows; Dickens, Woodside, and Westbury renamed Oaks. Allenby was converted back into semi-detached wards, in the form of East and West Hamlets, to house some of those from Easton Ward at Hortham. This wholesale move of patients and staff shook Brentry at a time when it was absorbed into Phoenix. It took several years for the staff to assimilate.

The closure of Hortham coincided with another change – the invention of the term Learning Disability. On the 25 June 1991 Steven Dorrell, Junior Minister of the Department of Health gave a speech to Mencap, in which he announced that the term preferred by the Department of Health for people with a mental handicap was now to be people with a learning disability. The other term that was used at that time by education, social services and many self advocacy groups was Learning Difficulties, but it was felt by health that this understated the issues involved.

Notes

[1] See DHSS: *Management Arrangements for the Reorganised National Health Service.* H.M.S.O. 1972; also *National Health Service Reorganisation Act 1973 (Chap.32).*

[2] *Bristol Evening Post* 29 May 1974

[3] *Bristol Evening Post* 11 June 1982

[4] *Bristol Evening Post* 30 Sept 1975

[5] *Bristol Evening Post* 21 Feb 1976 letter from R G Howse.

[6] *BRO:* 40795/2/S110 – D.M.T. 14 October 1976

[7] *BRO:* 40795/5/D21 – D.M.T. 10 Jan 1979

[8] *BRO:* 40795/5 – D21. D.M.T. minutes 14 Feb. 1979

[9] *BRO:* 40795/1 – M2 – D.M.T. – District Administrator paper dated 12 April 1976.

[10] *BRO:* 40795/1 – file D17/5

[11] *BRO:* 40795/1 – file D15

[12] *BRO:* 40795/5/D21 minutes 22 August 1978 and October 1978.

[13] *Report of the Committee of Enquiry into Mental Handicap Nursing and Care.* [Cmnd. 7468] London: HMSO. March 1979.

[14] Personal account.

[15] *BRO:* 40795/2 – S110 D.M.T. 14th October 1976.

[16] *BRO:*40795/4 – S102. Procedure dated 9 May 1978

[17] *BRO:* 40795/6

[18] *Western Daily Press* 3 November 1975, also in *Bristol* Evening Post 1 Nov.

[19] see details in local papers over next month.

[20] National Development Group for the Mentally Handicapped: *Mentally Handicapped Children: a Plan for Action.* Pamphlet 2, March 1977; also suggested in *Mental Handicap: Planning together.* Pamphlet 1, July 1976 and highly detailed description given in the *First Report 1976-1977* of the NDT.

[21] National Development Group for the Mentally Handicapped: *Residential Short-term Care for Mentally Handicapped People: Suggestions for Action.* Pamphlet 4, HMSO: May 1977

[22] National Development Group for the Mentally Handicapped: *First Report 1976-1977.* HMSO, 1978.

[23] *BRO:* 40795/2/S111

[24] *First Report 1976 – 1977.* Page 43.

[25] *BRO:* 40795/7 Medical Staff Advisory Committee minutes August 1978.

[26] South Western Regional Health Authority: *Improvements to Mental Handicap, Mental Illness and Geriatric Services.* January 1975

[27] *Bristol Evening Post* 15 October 1984

[28] *Bristol Evening Post* 23 November 1984

[29] *Bristol Evening Post* 3 December 1984

[30] Southmead Health Authority *Strategic Plan 1985-1995*

Phoenix NHS Trust

The Creation of Phoenix NHS Trust

Phoenix was the creation of the formidable South Western Regional General Manager, Ms Catherine Hawkins. For sometime she had been privately and publicly saying that the closure of mental handicap hospitals within the Avon area was well behind government targets and that a solution had to be found. The solution was Phoenix.

This was the time of NHS Trusts. The Government's solution to the problems of the NHS had been to reorganise it and to split commissioning from the provision of services. There were several waves of reorganisation, as more pressure was exerted to create the NHS Trusts. In the first wave, the Bristol and Weston Health Authority had split its provision of services into two Trusts, the Weston Trust and the large United Bristol Hospitals Trust, which contained the mental handicap services from Farleigh and Yatton. In the second wave of trust formation Southmead and Frenchay Health Authorities each decided to split off their health provision as a whole organisation - the Southmead NHS Trust which would have contained Brentry, and the Frenchay NHS Trust, which would have contained Stoke Park.

This was not to be. South Western Region informed Frenchay and Southmead that it would object to them forming Trusts if they included Mental Handicap Services within the Trust. In the end neither did. At the instigation of the South Western Regional Health Authority a new specialist Learning Disability Trust was created, taking over the learning disability services provided by Southmead and Frenchay Health Authorities and acquiring the learning disability services from the United Bristol Hospitals Trust. The new Trust was approved by the Minister in October. It came into being by means of a statutory instrument, *The Phoenix National Health Service Trust (Establishment) Order 1991,*[1] which came into force on the 1st November 1991 and set up the Phoenix NHS Trust on 1 April 1992, after a five month shadow period. Though the statutory instrument stated that the Trust's function

> shall be: a) own and manage hospital accommodation and services at Brentry … and associated hospitals; b) to manage community health services provided from Brentry Hospital.

The Trust spread its net much wider and did not use Brentry as its base. The Mental Handicap Unit managers of Southmead and Frenchay, Steve Strong and Liz Williams, joined the Executive Team working with David Selway who was appointed Chief Executive. David had been the director of the South Avon Housing Association before being appointed the Project Officer for the task of creating the new merged specialist health trust. The headquarters was set up at Stoke Park Hospital. Steve Strong left after about 18 months, and the finance officer Roger Moyse left afterwards to be replaced by Colin Hawkins in May 1995. Derek Smith was the first Chairman, having previously been chairman of the Bristol and Weston Health Authority.

There were some initial hiccups. Avon Social Services spoke little with Phoenix for more than a year, which made it difficult to plan or produce a well co-ordinated community service. The method of applying 'equal opportunities' to fit the old managers into the new middle management structure led to the failure of several of the people acknowledged to be the best managers in the old system to get a job in the new structure. This included managers from Brentry and Hortham. This did not help morale amongst the middle managers or on the wards. The consultant psychiatrists wrote a joint letter objecting to the formation of the trust. They said that the five year life expectancy of the trust made the work and disturbance of merging the three old areas into one unrewarding given the plan that the services then moved into another management structure. The new management team saw this letter as evidence of medical hostility to the new Trust. The appointment of the medical director was postponed until the rest of the executive team was properly established.

When Phoenix was first set up five management areas were created with Brentry part of North Bristol, with its manager Mrs Celia Powell in place by December 1991.[2] The hospital manager was Peter Conners, to be replaced by George Clemow the next year. In December 1993 the operations wing was restructured and the area system changed with the hospital system isolated from the community and 'therapeutic services'. Wyn Lewis became the manager of hospital services and Brian Currie became Nurse Manager for Brentry in 1994 after Vin Puttay had been in an acting role for a few months. There were further management changes at the end of 1995 when Phoenix split itself into Health and Social Care wings, with Wyn Lewis moving to become head of Social Care, but Brian Currie remained Nurse Manager at Brentry.

Though Phoenix was ostensibly set up to aid the closure of all the Mental Handicap Hospitals, Brentry was initially relatively untouched in that its closure was not planned in the first few years. In April 1992 there were 180 beds at Brentry. Robin Close had opened in April 1992. Brentry was the only old hospital site where Phoenix elected to purchase part of the site. It took on the ownership of the old Lower Village, though part was given up to build Repton House – a nursing home run by the Southmead Community Care Trust who ran most of the homes set up to close Hortham. The implication was for a long-term plan to continue to use the lower village after the long stay component of the hospital had closed. The upper village along with the main building were rented from the Regional Health Authority.

However in the first year there was a ward closure when Berkeley closed and Shannon ward moved into it, with the encouragement of the Mental Health Act Commissioners and Community Health Council who disliked the small heavily fenced compound attached to Shannon in its old location.

The next two hospital closures were Purdown in March 1992 and Farleigh in March 1993. After this the closure efforts were concentrated on Stoke Park which closed in March 1997, after several radical last minute changes in plans due to political changes. As part of the Stoke Park Closure, a ward of women and several individual patients were transferred from Stoke Park to Brentry, with many of the residents of Salisbury ward moved into Leese and Anderson.

Life under Phoenix

Life for residents at Brentry did improve with Phoenix. From its first prospectus the term used for patients was revised to Service Users, and so the inpatients at Brentry became Service Users with Learning Difficulties. The prospectus for Phoenix proposed to immediately implement "service user contracts" linked to the Individual Personal Plans, where each service user would be given a contract with the Trust, in which the service provided and its objectives would be stated. This was never implemented except in a highly modified form, but 'Individual Programme Plans'[IPPs] were introduced at Brentry for all the service users.

By the end of 1993 there was a user forum held at Brentry to enable the service users to comment on issues. Most of the forums across the service said that the hospital food was terrible, and the food improved. The service users were encouraged to vote in the general elections and there was a Voting Registration Roadshow held at Brentry in November 1995 to encourage the service users to register. This was a far cry from 20 years previously when no-one thought of the service users voting. They were being given a bigger voice.

In September 1995 the farm unit at Stapleton was developed into a Grounds and Gardens team to look after a range of homes and office bases, including Hanham Hall. This employed several Brentry service users. The day time therapy and activity services were formally split into Occupational Therapy and Day Services, with an improvement in the day-time activities for the service users at Brentry.

Phoenix also greatly improved the security on the site with outdoor video cameras and a daytime security officer, Dave, who became a popular figure amongst the staff and residents. The assaults of staff and residents by outsiders and the thefts from the site reduced, though it was still possible for a television to be removed from Jellicoe by a 'visitor' going up the back stairs.

At the end of 1996, Phoenix launched its own Service User Charter which promised fifteen things:

- You will have a key worker
- You will get food to eat, you can choose to eat:
    - healthy food
    - big or small helpings
- Staff will not shout or swear at you
- You will have enough staff to help you with your IPP Goals.
- You will have transport to help with your IPP Goals.
- Bosses will listen to you and think about what you say.
- If you use a wheel chair or are blind or deaf, you will get the help you need. You won't have to wait a long time for things.
- Phoenix places will have ramps and rails to help you get around.
- You will have good things to do during the day. Things that are not boring and make you feel good and show people that things you can do.
- You will get to learn new things or help to find a job if you want to.
- You will live in buildings and use places that are safe where you won't feel worried.
- You will have the same rights as other people so you can get to do the same things and use the same services.
- You will get the help you need to vote.
- You will have a say and get help to choose what you want to do.
- You can speak up if you are not happy or if there are things you would like to change.

This may not have been fully fulfilled but it was a complete change from the approach of earlier, and reflected the vogue for 'service user charters' in the rest of the NHS. Phoenix certainly did allow access to the bosses as the service users were welcomed to visit the trust headquarters: indeed one of the service users was well known for curling up and sleeping in the office of the Chief Executive.

The influx of new managers and new staff and patients led to a change in the staff attitudes and approaches to residents. However the wards still had large dormitories and there remained little privacy. In 1994 Phoenix set up an internal Healthcare Registration Team to inspect all of its wards and comment on how they could be improved. This was an attempt to rectify that deficit whereby the community homes were rigorously inspected in detail by an independent inspection team but hospitals were not. A complaints procedure was also set up which was adapted to be service-user friendly with visual symbols and audio tapes. The wards were renamed 'Homes' in October 1997, and the ward managers at Brentry were renamed home managers.

In 1996 Dr Sylvia Carpenter took over as Medical Director from Dr Jayewardene. As a result the medical cover for Brentry was reorganised. Dr Helen Sharrard became the sole consultant Psychiatrist for the long stay residents of Brentry though Dr Carpenter continued have her office on the site, as a member of the Bristol North CLDT and continued to admit patients for short-term Assessment and Treatment. Most of these admissions occurred on Shakespeare Ward, but some were admitted to Jellicoe and Colston.

In the 1997 election, there was a move to encourage the service users to vote. The service user forums initiated a series of information packs for staff to use to discuss issues with the service users. There were a series of workshops held to explore local topics such as transport.

The final closure plan

In June 1997 after Stoke Park closed, there were 128 residents in Brentry. The previous year the Avon Local Authority had been split into 4 smaller unitary authorities, Bristol, North Somerset, Bath and North East Somerset and South Gloucestershire. New relationships had to be forged and new agreements made. The closure of Stoke Park had been complicated by the plans made by Phoenix being taken over and revised at a late stage by Avon Health Authority. Of the 50 people planned to move out in 11 groups, 11 were not moved into planned new homes and only one group remained unchanged when Stoke Park finally closed. At the end of the closure of Stoke Park there was a severe financial crisis as Avon Health reduced the budget for Phoenix by three million pounds, a reduction of some 8%.

As part of the closure of Stoke Park the shrinking headquarters of Phoenix also moved across to Brentry and took over the Stables, including Shackleton as well as most of Baden Powell and the main house. For the first time in its life as an institution Brentry's managers were based on the site to the point that the Trust Board met there (except for the large AGMs that were held at Stapleton in the large New Friends Hall on the old Purdown site). Though in the past the senior managers had been based at Brentry the central management committee had never met there regularly – before 1948 these meetings were generally held in London and from 1949 to 1974 they had been held in central Bristol. Southmead Authority met there occasionally to show an interest, but this was the first time Brentry had been the base for a headquarters. It was now also the largest hospital for Learning Disability in Avon. The only other old long-stay hospital open was Hanham Hall on the other side of Bristol.

One consequence of the move of the headquarters to Brentry was a complete restructuring of the offices, with finance taking over the stable block. Baden Powell was used by the Chief Executive David Selway, and the Director of Operations, Liz Williams. The old Board Room, which was the main living room of the Burden's Flat, was taken over by Personel. As part of these changes the old dining room on the top floor of the stable block was closed and moved to a larger area beneath it. The old dining room had been one of the eccentricities of Brentry as the two ladies there had run a sit down restaurant service until the point that the room was closed. Menus were provided for each table and orders taken at the table, with the food brought to the person. It was not silver service, but it was a continuation of the old gentile style of life that had existed at Brentry, and which still provided a rewarding job in the small canteen. Its loss was a regret and a sign of the hustle of modern times.

Shortly before the move over of headquarters there was a sort out of many of the nooks and crannies in the main house. As part of this the 'gun room' – the small north west tower room – was cleared out and some of its cupboards opened to reveal guns that had been kept from the war, along with many of the old minute books of the HMC, which were transferred to the Record Office.

Avon now decided that it needed to close Brentry and Hanham at the same time. However the leader of the Avon management team who had overseen the closure of Stoke Park, Sue Prosser, had moved on just before Stoke closed, and so a new person Julie Sharma was appointed to lead the team after an interregnum held by Ian Maund. It was announced that Brentry would close by March 1999 at the latest, followed by Hanham Hall. The Commissioning team required that all the inpatients at both sites would be individually reviewed again and resettlement plans again be drafted for all of them by their social workers, building on the resettlement plans drawn up by the Phoenix resettlement team and social workers in 1995. In Brentry Bristol Social Services took the lead, reviewing all the residents who came from outside of Avon. This took about eight months of hard and heroic work, by the social work team and by the resettlement team appointed by Phoenix to help the process. The closure date for Brentry was by now clearly not going to be March 1999. Avon Health agreed in September 1998 for Bristol Social Services to take on the lead of the task of designing how to close Brentry with the Brandon Trust, preparing proposals for the resettlement. Brandon was the Community Care Trust that arose out of the closure of Farleigh. The proposal was for 58 new places to be built in 5 houses, ranging from a five bedded extension to an existing property, to a 16 bedded unit for the elderly.[3] There were not to be any isolated small units sitting in the community, but units reminiscent of the size being built in the 1970s (the 24 bedded units built in Wessex and at Hanham Hall), broken up into cloverleaf or similar designs. The service users were all given folders on 'My Life and Moving Home' to contain their photographic and written autobiographies and images of friends they knew at Brentry, as well as items related to their new homes.

During this time due to the old age of many of the residents, and some small scale discharge, Brentry had shrunk to only 75 residents in May 1999, living in seven wards ranging in size from six to 16 residents.

During the closure period though, Brentry did see some new building. Starting in May 1997, St Peter's Hospice was built on the site of the old Orchard and bowling green, entailing the demolition of the old laundry and other buildings that dated from the time of John Cave. St Peter's Hospice was completed at the end of 1998 and officially opened on 20 July 1999 (Figure 11.3).

During the closure period, Phoenix and Avon Health had several disputes. Following the General Election and change of government, Derek Smith did not have his term as chairman renewed a further time and he was replaced in December 1997 by Arthur Keefe, who had been the chairman of Avon Social Services, when Phoenix was formed. On 1st December 1998 the Chief Executive David Selway stood down due to the clashes between him and Avon Health Authority.

> My reason for leaving is that I feel the inaccurate, but negative, view held of me by certain key individuals in agencies outside of the Trust makes it impossible for me to serve the Trust effectively during what is a very important period for the service.[4]

Colin Hawkins took over for the final 16 months as both chief executive and finance officer. Wyn Lewis resigned at about the same time and died on 28 February 1999 from a heart attack. He was an able and well-liked manager who had devoted much of his life to the administration of the NHS. His death shook the service.

The end of 1998 also brought to a head the anxieties of the staff at Brentry. One long standing anxiety had been their future employment. In its initial period Phoenix had managed the staff who worked in the community care homes of the Brandon, Southmead and Frenchay Community Care Trusts. Nursing staff felt confident that that they had continued employment within the NHS though they were working for these Trusts. Then in September 1994 Avon Health formally considered a proposal to transfer the staff working in the community homes to the Community Care Trusts, outside of the NHS. Phoenix alerted the staff of this and the Avon Health Board meeting was attended by over a hundred protesting staff and television cameras. The decision was not taken, but the protest clearly soured relations between Avon Health and Phoenix. Phoenix's creation of a social care wing, and its taking over of the registered care homes managed by Southmead Community Care Trust, came out of the desire to keep employing the community care staff, who were becoming the majority of employees. By 1998 Phoenix was again on the defensive as Brandon and then the renamed Frenchay and Southmead Care Trust took over employing the

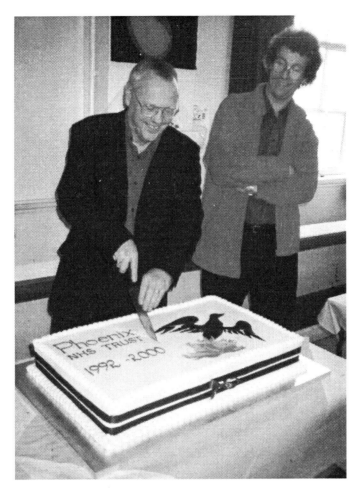

Figure 11.1: Cutting the cake to celebrate the achievements of Phoenix, 25 March 2000. Colin Hawkins cuts, whilst David Selway watches.

staff working in their homes in April 1999. At the end of 1998, the issue of the transfer of the remaining staff employed at Hanham Hall and Brentry came to a head. Brandon Trust argued whether it was obliged to take over the entire care staff working at Brentry on the same terms and conditions as they currently worked. In the end many staff sought redundancy on the closure of Brentry, and few transferred on the same terms and conditions as before.

Phoenix Trust was timetabled to close in April 2000, but by early 1999 it was still unclear what would happen to all its services. It was clear that Brentry and Hanham Hall would not close on schedule. Service users would be moving to new care homes with many of the care staff moving with them. What was being argued over was where the remaining health component would move – the retained services of Robin Close and a few other beds as well as the residential assessment and treatment service and the Community Learning Disability Teams with its specialist mental health service. What was clear was that all these services wanted to stay together. In March 1999 Avon Health decided that these services would all be transferred to the Bath and West Community Care Trust and not to the new Avon Mental Health Trust. The Bath and West Trust was based at St Martin's Hospital, in Bath and serviced the Bath, Devises and Frome areas, providing child health, old age and some learning disability services in Bath. It was however the only Community Care Trust in the Avon Area and it was recommended by an outside consultant Rob Greig that a Community Care Trust was where other learning disability services had felt happiest. By October 1999 the new Primary Care Trusts were being discussed and the long term future of the Bath and West Trust seemed less clear.

During all this the plans for the closure of Brentry continued apace as many of the managerial and other staff left to find alternative employment. The Health Authority formally published its proposal to close Brentry for consultation in October 1999. It was proposed that 58 of the residents would be moved into 5 purpose built homes, at least two of which would be nursing homes. By October 1999 four possible sites had been identified for these homes.

After a commemorative party held at Brentry on 26 March 2000 (Figure 11.1) Phoenix NHS trust was closed in April 2000 and its workings subsumed into Bath and West Community Care Trust. The service was split into two sub-units with Brentry and Hanham Hall being managed by one manager directly under the executive board, whilst the future specialist health services were managed separately. Most of this future service was kept as one managerial unit, which reduced the disturbance though there was a rearrangement of the middle management and the managers had to apply for new posts. This change did cause problems with morale as staff had to enable the closure of hospitals whilst applying for new jobs. Indeed several of the administrative staff did not know if they were being offered a post in the new Trust even a month before the closure of Phoenix.

As the management structure shrank, the local Community Learning Difficulties Team, the Bristol North team who covered the old Southmead area within Bristol, was able to move to old Baden Powell House and Ashwood – renamed Phoenix House and Lewis House (after Wyn Lewis).

The last patients left Brentry on 29 September 2000, leaving Hanham Hall as the last to close 7 weeks later. The gates and for sale signs went up in the upper village the next day. The medical records stored at Hanham Hall moved to old Anderson Ward. Phoenix House and Lewis House continued as the base of the North Bristol Community Learning Disability Team. Shakespeare, which had operated as the residential Assessment and Treatment service for the area was forced to close on 30 October on the undertaking that the money would be diverted into a new outreach service, but this failed to materialise and the money was 'lost'.

In April 2001 Bath and West Community Care Trust was dissolved and the services provided by it transferred to the new Bath and North East Somerset Primary Care Trust. In April 2002 the clinicians in the CLDT based at Phoenix House will have their management split between North and South Bristol and BANES Primary Care Trusts, with further reorganisations expected. The future of Robin Close is also being discussed. The service attempts to keep a motivated team to provide for People with a Learning Disability.

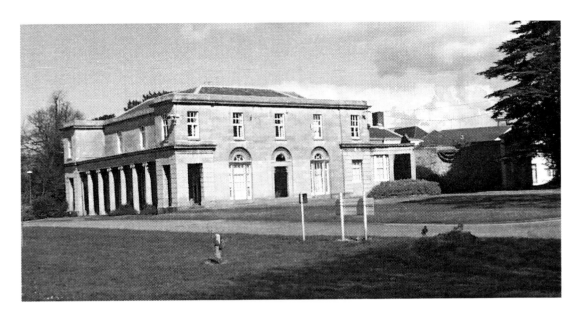

Figure 11.2: The main house October 2000

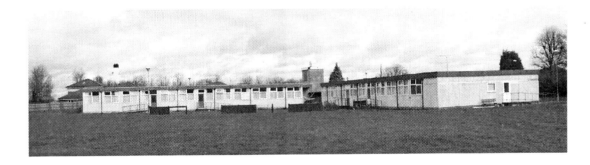

Figure 11.3: Willow and Blaise October 2000

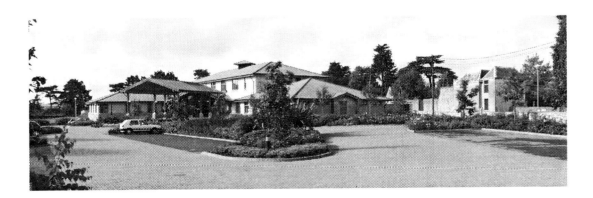

Figure 11.4: St Peter's Hospice and Boundary Cottage October 2000

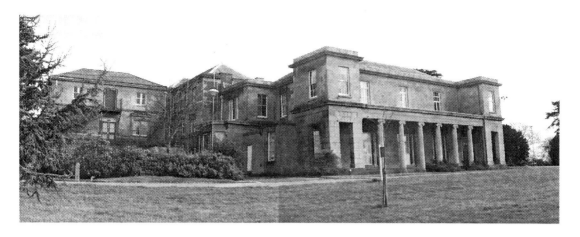

Figure 11.5: Brentry Main House October 2000

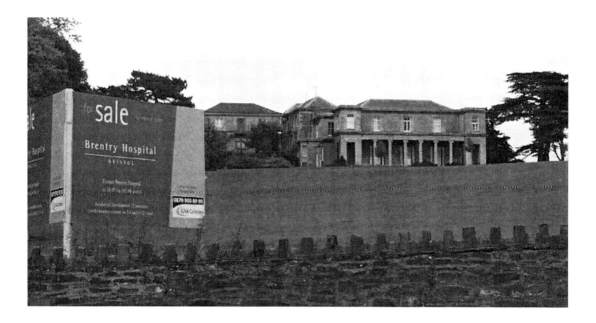

Figure 11.6: Hospital for sale.

Notes

[1] Statutory Instrument 1991 No 2385.
[2] Letter from Mrs Williams, dated 11 November 1991.
[3] Avon Health Authority: *Consultation Document on the Closure of Brentry Hospital, Hanham Hall, Berwick and Beesmoor.* Circa October 1999.
[4] Team Brief 2 December 1998

Epilogue

The contents of Brentry were auctioned in October and the main house and upper village sold to Countryside Properties South West Ltd for over 10 million pounds. It is planned to restore the old landscaping. All the buildings built after 1890 are being demolished apart from the 1904 kitchen block with 200 houses planned to be built mainly on the upper recreation ground, now called Royal Victoria Park (Figure 12.1).[1]

The main house is to be restored and the conservatory rebuilt. It is to be renamed Repton Hall. The stable block will also be restored and rebuilt, with new homes having gardens on the site of the 1930 laundry. Boundary Cottage is also to be rebuilt and restored as the triangular garden summer house but to function as a security lodge.

At the time of writing the buildings at Brentry are empty, except for those of the lower village which have been broken into and set fire to, despite being used as offices and a store for medical records. The smell of smoke still lingers after a year. The records have now been moved, filleted and the newer ones preserved. The older patient records have been burnt, except for a few sent to the Record Office. The Community Base has now become more used to operating without having the hospital next to it, as have the inpatient units in Robin Close. Some of the old residents look over the site and regret the loss of their activities there, though new ones are being found.

The estate is part of a cycle of life. It started as a home, and is again becoming a home, albeit for many more than originally. Similarly in its early life it saw the start of care for 'idiots and imbeciles' in charitable and private homes. The private sector is again the main provider of beds for people with 'learning disability'.

For the NHS the pace of life accelerates. The frequency of management reorganisation in the NHS has now increased to the point that the government appears to be talking of another major NHS management reorganisation, before the last one has been completed. The management of the Community Learning Disability Team staff will be separated out so that they are managed by three different Primary Care Trusts for the next year before being again reorganised. The new white paper, *Valuing People*, states that people with Learning Disability will now be fully integrated into the NHS. We can only hope that this intention becomes a reality and that they continue to obtain a service.

---

[1] *Western Daily Post* 10 July 2001. Page 21.

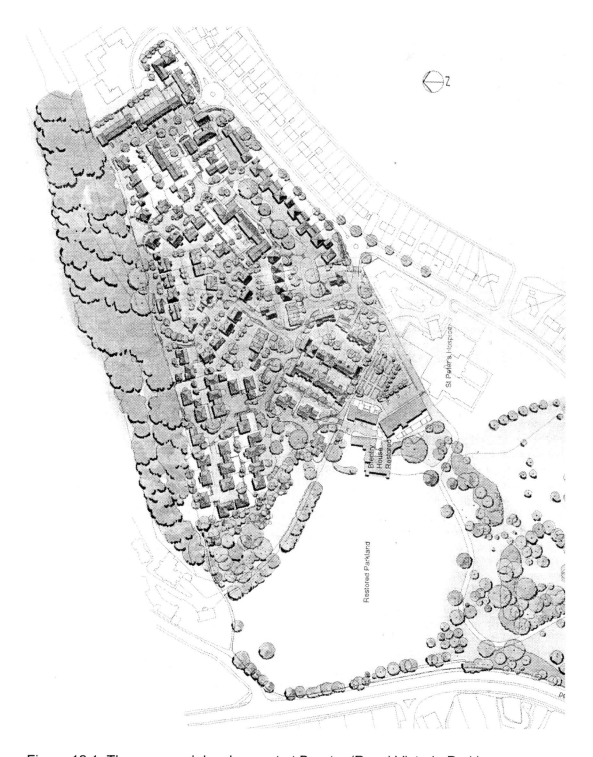

Figure 12.1: The proposed development at Brentry (Royal Victoria Park)

Appendix 1 – Names of the Wards

The names of the wards changed several times as wards were built, split and demolished. This is a listing of the wards.

Lower Village:

A:

    1899 opened as the first house for men

    1937 renamed Kipling

    1972 demolished

B:

    1900-1: built with a police station in basement and male receiving house on top floors.

    1937 renamed Baden Powell

    Being used at end of life as Sleeping accommodation only.

    1972 closed and reused as Occupational Therapy base

    1996 reused as offices (with basement for therapists)

    1999 renamed Phoenix House and used as Community Team Base.

C:

    1907 built.

    1937 renamed Haig

    1989 renamed Ashwood with admissions from Hortham.

    July 1995 closed to be used as staff training centre.

    1999 renamed Lewis House and used as CLDT base.

D:

    1900 built as a pair of semidetached cottages

    1937 renamed Allenby

    About 1989 divided back into two sides as East and West Hamlet

    May 1999 West Hamlet closed

    Sept 2000 East Hamlet closed

E:

    1900 built as a pair of semidetached cottages

    1937 renamed Shakespeare

    Used as Assessment and Treatment unit at end of life

    30 October 2000 closed after rest of site had closed.

Anderson:

    1972 built

    April 1999 closed

Leese:

    1972 built

    November 1999 closed

Upper Village:

<u>Stables:</u>

1899-1900 used as original retreat for women

1921 reused for a short time for last few female inebriates. Then converted to Workshops.

March 1933 part of ground floor reopened as Shackleton after conversion from old workshops.

July 1996 closed when converted into offices.

<u>A:</u>

1901 Originally built as women's infirmary

1937 renamed Dickens

1991 renamed Woodside

September 2000 closed when hospital closed.

<u>B:</u>

1900-1 built originally as two separate pairs of semidetached cottages for women

1926 infilled and merged into one block named B Block

1937 renamed Jellicoe

1955-9 split into Baldwin on ground floor and Jellicoe on top floor.

August 2000 Baldwin closed

September 2000 Jellicoe closed

<u>Warwick:</u>

1903 built as temporary ward to relieve overcrowding

March 1925 burnt down

1927 C block opened on site of Warwick

1937 C block renamed Wellington

1972 split into Westbury (upper floor) and Berkeley to accommodate women from Hortham.

1991 Westbury renamed Oaks

1992 Berkeley renamed Shannon.

August 1998 Oaks closed

May 2000 Shannon closed

<u>Reception House/ Hospital</u>

1903 Built as reception house for women to replace Horfield house.

1932 used for refractory patients

1933 used as hospital

1935 extended as Mather Jackson Hospital

Renamed Sick Ward and then Colston in the 1980s

September 2000 closed when hospital closed.

<u>Blaise:</u>

1971 built

March 1992 closed as ward – afterwards used for daytime activities

Charlton:
 1971 built
 1991 renamed Willow.
 September 2000 closed when hospital closed.

Hospital (Main house):
 March 1924 opened as Hospital when converted from staff accommodation.
 1933 converted into ward and renamed Darwin
 1991 renamed Shannon when received a ward from Hortham.
 July 1992 closed when Shannon name moved to Berkeley.
 Reused as offices.

Appendix 2 – Plans of the Main House

These plans come from Reptons 1802 publication, from the 1899 application for the house to become a reformatory, which shows the initial changes made, and then in 1922, a revised plan, which shows the additions to the second floor made after the 1904 fire.

Ground floor:

1802:

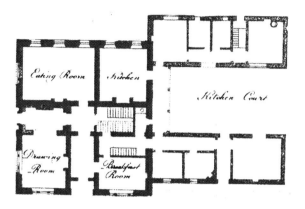

1899:

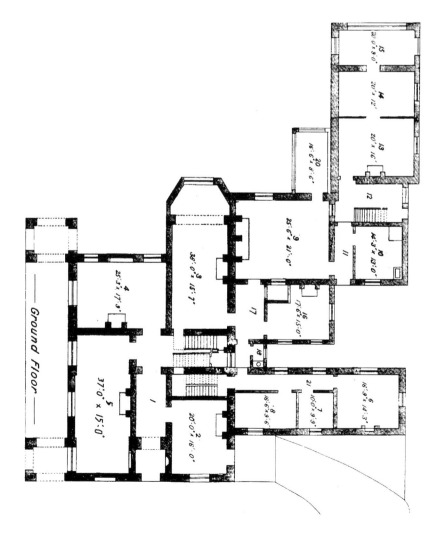

1922:

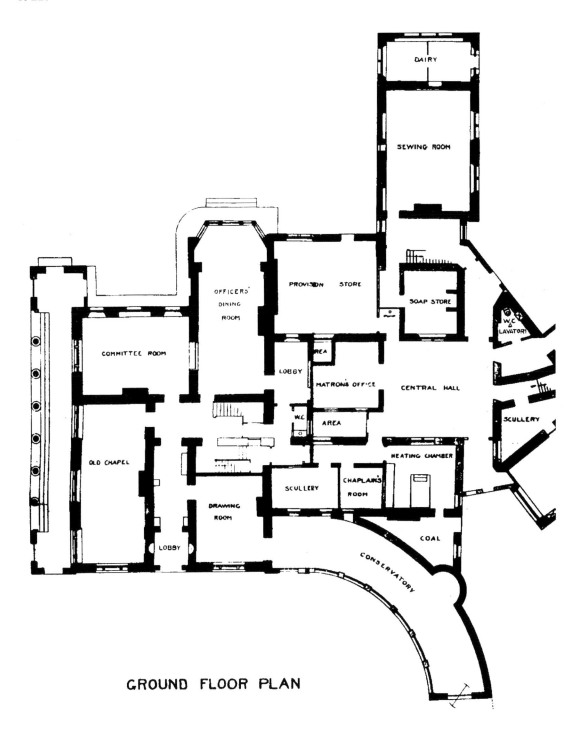

GROUND FLOOR PLAN

First Floor :

1899:

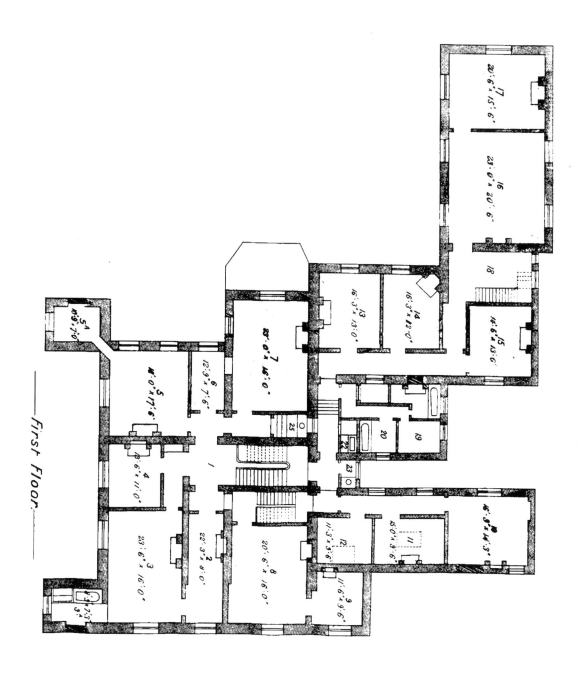

1922:

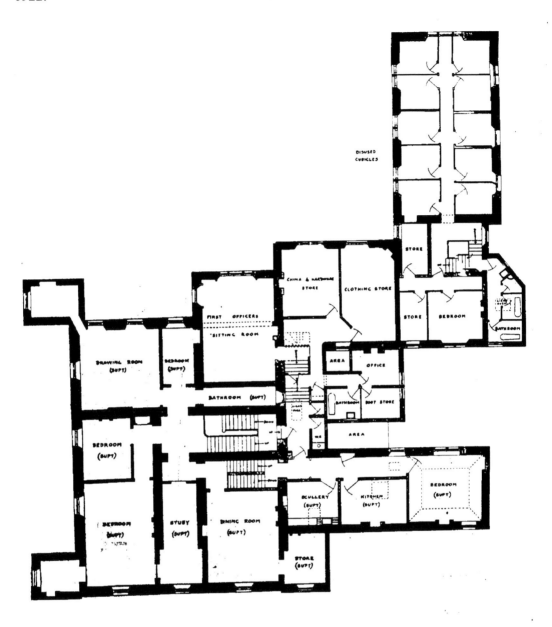

Second Floor:

1899:

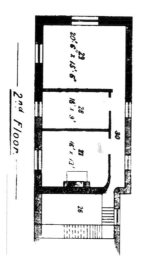

1922:

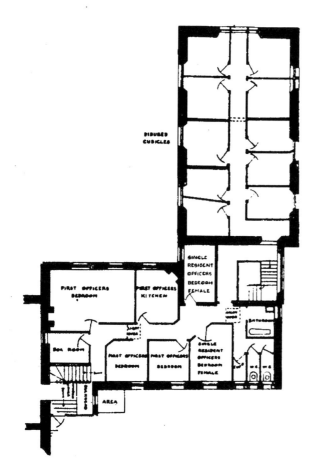

Appendix 3 – Statistics for inmates

1901 Census return for Brentry: RG13/ 2403 ff137-144

	Male	Female	Total
Total No Officers:	7	22	29
No in officers families	4	5	9
Other classes Inmates	21	98	119

Officers:

First Name	Surname	Sex	Relation	Marital status	Age	Occupation	Birthplace County
Harold Nelson	Burden	M	Head	Mar	41	Clerk in Holy Orders	Kent
Katherine Mary	Burden	F	Wife	Mar	43	Lady Superintendent	Yorks
Augusta	Garton	F	Aunt of above	Single	80	Living on own means	Yorks
Annie	Hopkins	F	Officer	Single	29	Assistant Matron	Somerset
Agnes	Cottle	F	Officer	Single	32	Assistant Matron	Wilts
Minnie	Bishop	F	Officer	Single	24	Day Attendant	Yorks
Charlotte	Buxton	F	Officer	Single	35	Day Attendant	Bristol
Ethel	Bye	F	Officer	Single	20	Day Attendant	Wilts
Louisa	Miller	F	Officer	Single	25	Day Attendant	Somerset
Marian	Tibble	F	Officer	Single	23	Day Attendant	Somerset
Amy	Willis	F	Officer	Single	27	Day Attendant	
Frederick	Bristow	M	Officer	Mar	39	Night Attendant	Wilts
Emma	Eeles	F	Officer	Single	30	Night Attendant	Oxfordshire
Clara	Gentle	F	Officer	Single	31	Night Attendant	Shropshire
Ellen	Miller	F	Officer	Single	35	Night Attendant	Ireland
Susan	Willmot	F	Officer	Single	23	Probation Nurse	Worcestershire
Ethel	Murray	F	Officer	Single	28	Garden Officer	London
Mabel	Murray	F	Officer	Single	29	Dairy Officer	London
Georgina	Keene	F	Officer	Single	38	Laundry Mistress	Wilts
Dorcas	Quick	F	Officer	Single	30	Kitchen Mistress	Devonshire
Alice Muriel	Rawson	F	Officer	Single	22	Store Keeper	Leicester
Elizabeth	Sawyer	F	Officer	Single	30	Assistant Laundry Mistress	Surrey
Mabel Norton	Steele	F	Officer	Single	21	Book Keeper	Bristol
Gladys	Williams	F	Officer	Single	32	Store Keeper (Clothing)	Cumberland?
William	Price	M	Officer	Mar	32	Police Constable	Gloucestershire
Joseph	Tilley	M	Officer	Single	26	Police Constable	Gloucestershire
Albert	Edwards And his wife	M	Officer	Mar	38	Gardener domestic	Gloucestershire
Fanny	Fox & her 3 sons	F	Officer	Mar	31	Gate Keeper	Gloucestershire
David	Pope & his wife & 2 children	M	Officer	Mar	36	Farm Bailiff	Worcestershire
James	Johns	M	servant	Mar	47	Well sinker	Herefordshire
Elizabeth	Pooley	F	servant	Single	49	Laundry Maid	Cornwall

Female Inmates – the names are given in census:

Age	Marital status	Occupation	Birthplace	Age	Marital status	Occupation	Birthplace
38	Mar	Charwoman	Birmingham	30	Mar		Cheshire
43	Mar		Birmingham	30	Mar	Dressmaker	Durham
45	Mar	Charwoman	Birmingham	41	Single	Servant (domestic)	Durham
47	Single	field worker	Birmingham	45	Mar	Laundry (Not Domestic)	Essex
49	Single	Hawker	Birmingham	45	Single		Essex
51	Single		Birmingham	48	Mar		Essex
25	Mar	Tailoress	Bristol	36	Mar		Flintshire
25	Single		Bristol	30	Single		Gloucestershire
34	wid	Cotton Spinner	Bristol	32	Mar	Tailoress	Hampshire
45	Mar	Cardboard Box Maker	Bristol	36	Mar	Charwoman	Hampshire
47	Wid	Fish Seller	Bristol	39	Mar	Servant (domestic)	Hampshire
44	Wid	Charwoman	Bucks	64	Wid		Hampshire
29	Single		Cheshire	34	Mar	Laundress	Hants

Age	Marital status	Occupation	Birthplace	Age	Marital status	Occupation	Birthplace
29	Wid	Servant (domestic)	Herefordshire	36	Mar	Laundress	Monmouthshire
41	Mar	Servant (domestic)	Hertfordshire	41	Mar		Monmouthshire
37	Mar		India	27	Mar		Norfolk
42	Wid		India	35	Single	Laundress	Norfolk
48	Wid	Hawker	India	36	Wid	field worker	Norfolk
30	Single	Baskle Woman	Ireland	45	Single	Laundress	Norfolk
41	Mar		Ireland	55	Mar		Norfolk
41	Mar		Ireland	27	Single	Kitchen Maid (not dom.)	Northumberland
41	Single		Ireland	35	Mar		Northumberland
30	Single		Isle of Man	35	Single	Rope Factory Worker	Northumberland
34	Mar	Artist's Model	Isle of Wight	41	Mar	Servant (domestic)	Northumberland
43	Mar		Kent	54	Mar		Northumberland
37	Single		Leicester	48	Wid		Nottingham
44	Single	Charwoman	Leicester	31	Mar	field worker	Oxfordshire
41	Mar	Laundress	Lincoln	37	Mar	Nurse (domestic)	Plymouth
40	Single	Laundress (Not dom.)	Liverpool	40	Mar	Cotton Spinner	Scotland
51	Mar		Liverpool	42	Mar	Shirt Machinist	Scotland
34	Single	Bar maid	London	42	Single	Cotton Spinner	Scotland
36	Wid		London	68	Mar	Domestic Servant	Scotland
37	Mar		London	36	Mar		Somerset
38	Mar		London	49	Mar	Charwoman	Somerset
38	Mar		London	31	Mar	Hawker of artificial flowers	Staffordshire
38	Mar		London	34	Mar		Staffordshire
42	Mar		London	46	Mar	Potter	Staffordshire
45	Wid	Charwoman	London	43	Mar	Laundress	Suffolk
46	Mar	Field Worker	London	31	Mar		Surrey
47	Mar		London	47	Mar	Parlor maid (domestic)	Surrey
48	Wid	Corset Maker	London	24	Single	Servant (domestic)	United States
50	Mar		London	45	Mar	Cook (domestic)	Warwickshire
57	Mar		London	70	Wid	Needlewoman	Warwickshire
40	Single	Milliner	London?	36	Mar	Hawker	Worcestershire
30	Mar	Laundress	Middlesex	28	Mar		Yorkshire
33	Mar	Laundress (Not dom.)	Middlesex	31	Mar		Yorkshire
44	Mar		Middlesex	48	Single	Charwoman	Yorkshire
45	Mar	Laundress	Middlesex				
26	Single	General Servant (dom.)	Monmouthshire				
29	Mar	Charwoman	Monmouthshire				
35	Mar		Monmouthshire				
35	Single	Barmaid	Monmouthshire				

Male Inmates: -again names and further birth details given in census

Age	Marital status	Occupation	Birthplace	Age	Marital status	Occupation	Birthplace
31	Single	Shoe Maker	Bristol	26	Single	Chimney Sweep	Middlesex
34	Single	House Painter	Bucks	29	Single	General Labourer	Nottingham
33	Mar	Watchmaker	Carmarthenshire	60	Single	General Labourer	Nottinghamshire
39	Single	Hammerman	Essex	44	Mar	China Riveter?	Somerset
31	Single	Dealer in Rags etc	Herefordshire	35	Single	Keysmith	Staffordshire
30	Single	General Labourer	Hertfordshire	71	Mar	Saddler	Staffordshire
40	Mar	Boatman	Kent	41	Mar	Fisherman	Sussex
49	Mar	Seaman	Kent	27	Single	General Labourer	Worcestershire
49	Single	General Labourer	Kent	36	Single	General Labourer	Worcestershire
22	Single	General Labourer	London	47	Mar	Farmer	Worcestershire
33	Single	General Labourer	London				

Royal Victoria Home (Horfield, Prison Road) RG13/ 2398 ff107 – lists only two officers as resident.

Name	Relationship	Mar.	Age	Occupation	Birthplace
Rosina Broom	Officer in charge	Single	34	Senior attendant	Bristol
Elizabeth Kirby	Servant	Single	47?	Cook (domestic)	Gloucs, Charfield

Costs of Brentry in 1907[*]

	Av No	Lic	Staff Exp	Inmate Exp. (eg provis)	General expenses	Manage-ment exp.	Less in-mate income	Actual weekly cost
†E Harling	223	209f	3/8½	4/11¾	1/5¾	1/3	½	10/2¼
†Ackworth, Yorks	65	90f	4/3	4/11½	1/9¼	1/3½	1/2¼	11/2¼
†Lewes	131	150f	3/11½	5/1½	1/11½	1/3¾	1/1½	11/3½
†Midland	31	57f	4/3½	5/4	2/0¾	1/7_	1/6½	11/9¾
†RVH Horfield.	10	20f	4/7	4/11¼	2/4¾	1/5½	1/5	11/11_
Brentry	219	240	4/9	5/4½	2/3½	0/5¾	0/3	12/7
Langho Lancs	138	185f	5/11¼	4/9¼	2/8½	1/1_	2/0½	12/7
Duxhurst Reigate	10	32f	5/10¾	6/9½	1/4¼	1/11	0/2	15/9½
Farmfield Horley	105	113f	5/1_	5/9½	4/4	1/7½	0/0½	16/10
Cattal Yorks	63	80	9/1¼	6/1¾	7/3½	1/10	½	23/2½

† Operated by the *National Institutions*

Interestingly, the cost given for Brentry for 1907 in the Brentry Annual report for 1920 is 13/1½d per inmate per week, which is higher than that given by the Inspector.

---

[*] Annual Report of Inspector of Certified Reformatories 1907: 1908 xii 1107 [Cd.4342]

Statistics for Inebriates in Brentry (excludes readmissions)[*]

Year	Admissions during year (including transfers)			‡National New Admission	Number at end of year		
	Males	Females	Total	Total	Male	Female	Total
1899			46	88			?
1900	16	86	102[♦]	144	13	68	81
1901	33	133	171[○]	204	34	163	197[§]
1902	34	73	107	278			?
1903	30	77	107	298	52	147	199
1904	37	63	100	418	63	132	195
1905	87	34	121	443	100	98	198
1906	81	35	116	404			209[§]
1907	46	61	107	493	134	92	226[§]
1908	34	41	75	262	109	100	209[§]
1909	46	33	79	277	82	102	184[§]
1910	57	30	87	327	103	76	179
1911	61	37	98	339	129	83	212
1912				305	126	78	204[§]
1913	76	30	106	310	131	70	201
1914					123	75	198[§]
1915					78	141	219
1916	>6	>30	>36		36	108	154
1917					11	49	77
1918					1	18	19
1919	-	1	1		-	6	6
1920	-	4	4		-	3	3
1921	-	1	1		-	0	0

[♦] includes 18 admitted as Retreat in Ann report of Inspector of reformatories - wardens report for year says 75 admitted

[○] total includes 6 admitted as Retreat, but these are not included in sex breakdown.

[§] numbers in residence for return not of 31 Dec but within 3 months

[‡] committals to reformatories as given in the annual reports of the Inspector under the inebriate acts.

[*] Source: Admissions: annual report for Brentry for 1911, and the Annual report of Inspector for 1899 and for retreat admissions; also annual reports (and where not available quarterly reports) for numbers remaining. Please note the Annual reports seem to apply only to reformatory cases.

Statistics for Mental Defectives

Year ending March:	Patient statistics (all male) for year 1 April - 31 March			
	Admitted	Discharged/	On leave on 31	Inpatients on 31
1918	108	5		**103**
1919	48	40	2	**109**
1920	87	12	-	**184**
1921	65	22	7	**220**
1922	70	49		**228**
1923	20	23		**220**
1924	43	22		**231**
1925	64	9	12	**278**
1926	45	40	17	**279**
1927	52	20	23	**304**
1928	71	12	33	**347**
1929	28	42	35	**330**
1930	42	40	37	**330**
1931	25	35	36	**314**
1932	41	26	41	**321**
1933	47	28	48	**336**
1934	63	40	51	**357**
1935	48	67	62	**333**
1936	98	41	88	**371**
1937				
1938	37	28	94	**396**
1939				
1940	60	45	54	**405**
1941	31	16	56	**415**
1942 ♦	33	35	58	**408**
1943			62 ○	**393**
1944				**378**
1945	39	9		**389**
1946	57	27	91	**420**
1947	28		78	**427**
1948	20		71	**431**

♦ data not in Annual report but from Board of Control report for June 1942, and covers 13 months.

○ from Board of Control report 17 March 1943

Use of beds at Brentry for Mental Deficiency by Councils.

Source: Annual reports for year, bed numbers is number of beds occupied plus those on leave.

	1920	1931	1941
Major users (use 10 beds or more)	34 Lancashire	51 Middlesex	63 Monmouthshire
	26 NIPRCC	48 Monmouthshire	56 Middlesex
	18 Middlesex	44 Gloucester/shire	54 Gloucester/shire
	12 London	26 Kent	32 Swansea
		21 West Ham	26 West Ham
		19 Birmingham	24 Salop
		17 Reading	22 Wolverhampton
		10 Buckinghamshire	20 Birmingham
			16 Worcestershire
			15 Kent
			13 Newport (Mon.)
			12 Nottinghamshire
			11 Eastbourne
			10 Cornwall
			10 Warwick
Total of major users	90 used by 4 users	236 used by 8 users	384 used by 15 users
Other beds	94 used by 40 users	116 used by 27 users	95 used by 31 users
Totals	**184 used by 44 users**	**352 used by 35 users**	**479 used by 46 users**

Statistics within the NHS

Rather oddly it is very difficult to discover what were the inpatient statistics for Brentry for most of its time in the NHS. This was partly complicated by a flood in the cellars that destroyed many files and records. However these are the figures that are known.

Year ending March:	Patient statistics (all male) for year 1 April - 31 March			
	Admitted during year	Discharged/ Transferred/ died etc during year	On leave on 31 March	Inpatients on 31 March (31 December from 1986)
1949				
1950				
1951	27	34	67	**416**
1952				
1953	36	42	36	**419**
1954	33	37	18	**427**
1955	27	24	17	**429**
1956	26	20	19	**431**
1957	17	22	16	**432**
1966				**440***
1971				**420***
1974				**398***
1980				**362**[†]
1985				**241**[†]
1987				**207**
1988				**205**
1989				**192**
1990				**170**
1991				**190**
1992				**160**
1993				**153**
1994				**149**
1995				**144**
1996				**128**
1997				**121**
1998				**97**
1999				**61**

* Month of year for which this number applies not known – numbers given in H.M.C. 14 Jan 1974

[†] registered bed numbers given in regional year book of this year

Appendix 4 – a 1929 account of Mental Deficiency Colonies

The deficits in the quality of the accommodation and staffing at Brentry in the 1920s need to be set against the idealistic comments of the period. The Boards of Control and of Education set up a Mental Deficiency Committee to review the care of the mental defective. The report was published in 1929 and reassured the public on the care available within institutions. Its idealised description of life in the mental deficiency colonies now makes interesting reading, especially as it implied that only a few failed to be up-to-date. So this is what it was really like in the colonies?:[*]

We propose ...to describe the best and the most modern type of institution ... In reading this description then it must never be forgotten that there are some institutions where the arrangements for classification are defective and those for teaching inadequate, where the staff is insufficient both in number and quality, where occupations present little variation and are confined to the routine work of the institution, and where provision for recreation and occupation during the patients' free time is quite inadequate. To those responsible for these institutions we hope the following description will be both an incentive and an ideal.

The happiness of Institution life.

19.   Perhaps the first lesson to be learnt from up-to-date institutions and one which it is important that the public should know and appreciate is that, contrary to what is frequently supposed by those who have no knowledge of them, they are happy places for those detectives who are fortunate enough to get into them. This happiness is certain for those who are admitted while still children, but it is true that contentment, happiness and even obedience do not come so easily to those detectives whom society has failed to rescue until their outlook and nature have been impaired by bad associations, evil doings and unrestricted licence. Up-to-date institutions are not merely places of detention. They are also schools, colonies, places of training, hospitals and homes where every effort is made to give each patient the fullest possible life. Though a great deal of work is done inside them, recreation holds a no less important place. Though many of the patients will remain in them all their lives (and the large majority will be glad and happy to do this), yet there is the spirit of hope strongly present for all those mentally able to appreciate it. Every effort is made with the higher grade patients so to teach and train, so to stabilise them, so to increase gradually the responsibility placed on them, that they may be socialised and find their way back to the world to live there a happy useful life in some lowly occupation fitted to their capacity. The ordinary adult defective has a poor time in the outside world. There is liberty it is true, but in many cases it is liberty only to get into mischief. In thinking of the detectives in an institution we should clear our minds of a good deal of false sentiment. In the institution they have care, good food, easy occupation without overwork or driving, plenty of recreation, no worry because of real wrong-doing, and above all the feeling of equality, the feeling that they are as capable or even a little more capable than their neighbour. Outside, there is the constant feeling of inferiority, the knowledge that they will be the first to lose their job if employment gets slack. Most of those who come to an institution with a bad record, do, in the atmosphere they find there, quickly settle down. One of the chief causes of happiness or unhappiness is the opinion of the herd on the individual member of it. A defective in the outside world is never allowed to believe in himself, he has perpetual past failure to discourage him, he has not had in any well-behaved sphere a situation he could control. Often wrong-doing is the only course that appears to offer any kind of situation he can control, and he takes it for the satisfaction of success. On the other hand, an institution for detectives is, for the great majority of its patients, a very happy place. It gives them care suited to their needs and employment -regulated according to their ability.

The institution has two great advantages to offer its patients. One is that the conditions of living and the relief from care are a great improvement on life outside ; the other is the spirit inside the institution. Everyone is there to learn, to be trained, to be helped and if at first

[*] *Report of the Mental Deficiency Committee, being a Joint Committee of the Board of Education and Board of Control. Part III - the Adult Defective.* London: H.M.S.O., 1929. Pages 21 – 25.

the newcomer does not appreciate this, the " esprit de corps " amongst - those already there quickly makes it clear.

The modern institution is generally a large one, preferably built on the Colony plan, taking detectives of all grades of defect and all ages. All, of course, are properly classified according to their mental capacity and age. The Local M.D. Authority have to provide for all grades of defect, all types of case and all ages, and an institution that cannot or will not take this case for one reason and that case for another is of no use to the Authority. An institution which takes all types and ages is economical because the high grade patients do the work and make everything necessary, not only for themselves, but, also, for the lower grade. In an institution taking only low grades the whole of the work has to be done by paid staff; in one taking only high grades, the output of work is greater than is required for the institution itself, and there is difficulty in disposing of it. In the all-grade institution on the other hand the high grade patients are the skilled workmen of the colony, those who do all the higher processes of manufacture, those on whom there is generally a considerable measure of responsibility; the medium grade patients are the labourers, who do the more simple routine work in the training shops and about the institution; the best of the lower grade patients fetch and carry, or do the very simple work like cleaning spoons or polishing the floors, and quite the lowest grade are the drones for whom all the others work. One of the aims of the modern institution is to make and keep in repair everything it needs for its own use, such as clothing, boots and furniture. In most cases too it constructs, by its own labour, the smaller building additions that are necessary. It is this variety of occupation that enables it to find useful work for all grades of detectives.

Trade Training.

20.   In the case of the majority of the recognised trades, each shop is in charge of a skilled tradesman who had learned his trade before he began work for detectives ; but his skill in teaching defectives he has to gain by experience at the actual work. This applies also to many of the female staff teaching, for instance, tailoring, dressmaking, laundry work. There has been nowhere any course of training for the tradesmen, either in their trade as applied to detectives or in general methods of teaching. Recently, however, the Medico-Psychological Association has fundamentally altered the syllabus of training for its certificate for those nursing the mentally defective, and the trade teachers will now be able to prepare and enter for examinations each in his own speciality.

In certain of the less highly skilled occupations the instruction is however usually given by one of the nurses or attendants who has learned the work in the institution. This applies almost always to such occupations as rug making, all the various forms of raffia and cane work, leather work, much of the needlework and such things as paper bag making and some of the simpler forms of brush-making.

Forms of work by Defectives for use in Institutions.

21.   The usual occupations may now be described in somewhat more detail. Tailors' shops make all the male clothing and the staff uniforms. Most of the higher grade patients are allowed the opportunity of selecting the cloth for their own suits or frocks. All patients except those of the lowest grades have their own clothes marked with their own names and reserved for their especial use. This principle. is just as important for the self-respect of the patient as the provision of towels, flannels, brushes and combs, each marked with the individual patient's name and used only for that patient, is vitally necessary for the sake of cleanliness and the prevention of infection. Needlework rooms make all the underclothing for both sides of the institution, the women's frocks and staff uniforms, and knit by machine all socks, stockings and jerseys that are required. The. present opinion is that all these shops should be as fully equipped as possible with machines. To make a garment by hand is tedious and monotonous, whereas with a machine a girl can make a dozen shirts instead of one in the same time and has the satisfaction of a pile of work done. The principle of increasing the use of machinery is of general application to all trades; the old days when the chief aim was to give the defective a job which would keep him or her quiet as long as possible are dying out. Repair work to clothes and house linen is exceedingly heavy. Sometimes this is carried out in separate shops, sometimes in the same shops as the new work. Most institutions repair all their own boots and shoes, and many of them make all the new boots and shoes and slippers. The carpenter's shop undertakes all repairs of furniture and carpenters' repairs to the buildings and estate, and all the new furniture required should be made in this shop. Some institutions do their own printing and binding, others make and repair their own tinware. Some have weaving shops in which the women's frock material,

both washing and serge, is made as well as some of the men's cloth, Oxford shirting, quilts, towelling, blankets and sheeting. Most of these weaving shops begin work with the ordinary wooden hand loom, then add the semi-automatic iron loom, and after that some power looms. These latter make a great difference to the output.

Gardening is done both by male and female patients, and the larger institutions have farms which employ a good deal of male labour. Male patients are also employed at painting the institution, bricklaying and concrete work. Laundry, kitchen and house work employ many of the female patients, a few can be used as staff mess-room maids and many are glad to be allowed to help, of course under supervision, in caring for the lower grade children.

Most institutions also carry on trades for the making of goods which can be sold, such as brushes, both drawn and pitched, baskets, hampers, basket work chairs, yarn, wool-bordered and wool rugs, made both on looms and frames and by hand, carved wooden goods, straw hats, toys, both wooden and stuffed, cane chairs, trunks, etc. There are also the more fancy trades, such as lace making, leather work of all kinds, raffia work, tapestry weaving, the knitting of woollen coats, jumpers and frocks, glove making, fancy needlework and embroidery, and many of the female patients prefer, in their leisure time, to do crochet, lace and drawn-thread work, often of a very high class.

Diet.

22. The diet of the patients deserves and receives the greatest consideration; but this question has been so recently and exhaustively studied in "The Report on the Dietary in Mental Hospitals", prepared by a Committee appointed by the Board of Control, that there is no need to go into it here. It is enough to say that in the best institutions the recommendations of this Committee have been widely adopted.

Recreations.

23. It is the usual custom to give all patients who work weekly pocket money. In the modern institutions as much attention is paid to the amusements of the patients as to their work. As already mentioned Guide Companies and Scout Troops are the rule, and as a result of the intensive training that is possible at an institution these companies frequently obtain good places in competition at the local rallies. Summer camps under canvas for some of the patients are a great treat. The majority of the patients, either because of their own weaknesses, or from the type of their homes, are unable to go home for a holiday, and the seaside home connected with the institution enables them to get a change, where more liberty and freedom can be granted than is always possible in the institution itself. Cricket, hockey and football matches for interhouse shields and against outside teams are the rule, and it is becoming common to enter a team in the local football league. Physical exercises and gymnasium work for both sexes are excellent, and athletic sports are regularly held. Among indoor recreations dancing holds the first place with the girls and every day room should have its own gramophone, and if possible a piano. Amongst the boys billiards or bagatelle are more popular, and the numerous competitions amuse not only those actually playing, but a big circle of others who are content to watch and smoke. Weekly or fortnightly cinema shows are greatly enjoyed, and in addition there are mixed whist drives, dances and frequent concerts and entertainments, both by professional and amateur companies. Defectives themselves love dressing up and all kinds of dramatic work, and most institutions make a point of giving plays in which all the performers are patients. Some of them are very elaborate and are attended and paid for by crowded audiences from outside. The institution magazine edited by patients is a recent feature, and there are several brass and other bands composed almost entirely of patients who, besides playing for the entertainment of the inmates, get paid for outside engagements. Walking out on parole is a much prized privilege, but it is wise to send out three together rather than two.

Discipline.

24. The methods of discipline in an institution for detectives are somewhat like those of a big family. Though there will always be a minority of difficult and unstable cases which will need all the wisdom and judgement of those in authority and all the discretion and tact of the staff, the majority of detectives are easy, kindly people to manage, just like so many children with rather short memories. A simple joke will frequently help more than scolding, and praise, and still more praise for work well done, is more effective than anything else. Before admission to an institution a defective has not had much praise as a rule. When these methods fail the taking away of small privileges, like loss of parole, loss of pocket money, boots to wear instead of shoes, missing

some treat like a party, a dance or an entertainment, can be used. Corporal punishment is illegal, and rightly so, and the cutting out of necessary food has been abandoned. In the unstable hysterical type of patient, bed for a day or two has a quietening and stabilising effect, and some girls, when they know an attack is coming on, will ask to be allowed to stop in bed.

Appendix 5 – An account from 1945

A speech by Dr Mason has survived. Who he talked to is not known, but the paper seems to give an honest and critical view of the working of Brentry just prior to the new NHS and the deficiencies both in its staff, and of the mental deficiency act. Therefore the talk is reproduced in its entirety:

<u>The Mental Defective Delinquent in Institutional Care</u>* 5/2/45

Mr. Chairman,

Before I had committed my preliminary browsings on this subject to paper I was favoured with a preview of Dr. Benjacer's notes and was at once struck by the similarity of his views with my own. As the class of work he and I are engaged in is, I believe, very similar, this must mean that we are both right. Despite this preview then, I am pleading justification for submitting what may appear a paraphrase of the paper you have just heard.

The Mentally defective delinquent of near adult or adult life age is most commonly discovered in the course of police-court proceedings (Sect.8) [*which allowed magistrates to make an order sending a convicted person to a mental deficiency institution*]. Many so discovered must constitute the leakage of unsatisfactory early ascertainment, largely in the hands of the education authorities, though some are detectives known since childhood as such, perhaps dealt with in special schools, but subsequently left under loose supervision or without any, until placed under an Order, generally through possible police charges being dropped in favour of Sect.6 procedure at a more advance age [*section 6 permits judicial authority to commit a person of an institution if he felt it desirable in the person's interests*]. Others reach prison or a Borstal before ascertainment, when they become certified under Sect.9 [*by which they can be transferred from prison to an institution*].

The majority of delinquent defectives, certified in or after adolescence are feeble-minded, there are some moral defectives. The imbecile delinquent is not so common, having been obvious at an earlier age and, when presented in adult life, is generally so through the dropped charge process under Sect.6.

The comparatively high present day figure of mental detectives from these sources is, I think, the result of a higher speed communal activity all round, war time facilities for the commission of offences (both revealing the incompetence and impulsiveness of the defective more obviously) and an improved diagnosis by the court medical and lay advisers. There is perhaps too, a tendency to apparent leniency within statutory requirements which may cause a Magistrates bench to search more diligently for an alternative to punishment. Dr. Benjacer has suggested the question whether too broad an interpretation is not current. Indeed some Magistrates both on bench and Committees do show occasionally by their actions and conversation that they regard the Mental Deficiency Acts as mildly penal in character and the Colony as a modified prison or reformatory. Others still more unsatisfactorily confuse it with Poor Law administration. The question "what's he in for" is too often asked by who should know better. Perhaps our Magistracy is too often a reward for long service in local government without regard to intellectual equipment.

At a Colony accommodating solely male defectives, of ages at or over adolescence, reviewing the last 157 new admissions, 80 have been certified under Sect. 6 of whom half could probably equally well have been dealt with under Sect.8, 49 were Police convictions (Sect.8), 21 came from penal establishments (Sect.9) and the balance of 7 by Varying Order. Thus 74% are actual delinquents though only 49% have been found guilty of an offence in a Court of Law.

The Offences most usual are larceny, housebreaking, interferences with children, indecent exposure, sexual and common assaults in that order. I agree with Dr.Benjacer that when one learns the details, in many instances the charges seem trivial, but real serious dangers to the public are often removed by the reception of these patients. There is a capacity for public danger, not merely public nuisance, in the defective.

Of the 70 cases under Sects. 8 & 9, 28 are feeble-minded with mental ages of 9 upwards, 35 are feeble-minded with mental ages from 6 to 9 and 7 are imbeciles with mental

---

* *BRO*: 40686/B/GF/1g

ages from 3 to 6. The moral defective seldom appears, certifying doctors seem uneasy about this class and unwilling to use the designation. As the legal definition provides that there is feeble-mindedness present in any case it is natural to avoid a gratuitous complication. The moral defective whose feeble-mindedness is not quite apparent avoids the M. D. Acts in this way. He may belong to a group in which are also the psychopaths and the constitutional psychic inferiors.

Dr. Benjacer has referred to the undesirable habit of minor officials of the public authorities, who insure themselves against unpleasantness or difficult explanations by misleading the patient and often his relatives by assurances that the detective is only going to a school for a year where he will learn this or that, and be faithfully sent home to live happily ever after. Alternatively that he has received a one year sentence at a nice new kind of prison, with the same rosy future attached.   These assurances are so common as to be usual and undoubtedly add to the duration of an adverse reaction in the patient after arrival. They cannot be too strongly condemned.

In practically every Colony at the present time, the high-grade new arrival receives almost unwarned the shock of propinquity with obvious mental abnormals.   Complete segregation of other than idiots is usually impracticable. This shock Is probably not much less than that likely in a normal person so situated. When mislead by false assurances immediately before arrival, the reaction is manifestly deepened.

Berry and Gordon* have used McDougall's grouping into the self-abasing type and the self-assertive type in explaining conduct development in the defective. Such an introduction into Institutional care increases the anergic dispondency of the former type and precipitates refractoriness in the latter.

The attitude of the parents is interesting. Practically every case of parental hostility I have experienced has come from the parents or patients who belong to the aggressively undisciplined assertive type, usually those certified in connection with delinquency.   Real incapacity to understand is met with chiefly from parents who are themselves subnormal. A truthful and frank visitor to the home can usually clear this up. Occasionally aggrieved and hostile parents have a local councillor at their call. When such a combination occurs, plain statements of fact are seldom overruled, but it is generally best to refer such cases to the Board of Control. This last situation no doubt seldom bothers the superintendent of Colonies managed by the local authority itself, but it does occur quite frequently in independent or voluntary institutions.

Parents and others frequently write unsuitable and inflammatory matter to the patient as well as to the medical superintendent. It is better to induce the writers by personal efforts to desist from this practice rather than exercise the power of suppression of such correspondence. In these cases it is nearly always intensely difficult to obtain the patient's real trust and co-operation, though the natural cunning of the defective often succeeds in an effective pretence of this.

Under present day conditions. only slightly modified by the recent Rushcliffe wage award, difficult labour conditions make it necessary sometimes to retain men on the staff whose outlook, understanding and willingness is far from satisfactory. This type of "male nurse" (I use the term in inverted commas) may league himself consciously with the mischief-making resentful patient and thereby do untold harm. The higher grade delinquent defect is a very stubborn wrong-doer; he enters a Colony, open in character, where no facilities for strict segregation exist, is quick to sense an undisciplined slackness amongst the staff, or as quickly recognises the weak, foolish or discontented individual among the staff. There is an approach, a mutual interchange of grievances, a sense of kinship. Thus real difficulties can arise, much mischief can be done. The cause may be hard to fathom. Some years ago a group of delinquent high grade patients spotted a regular breech of rules by certain male nurses whose discontent had induced deliberate laxity of duty. The result was a series of burglaries in the district carried out by three or four lads almost nightly while supposed to be safely in bed. On discovery these patients were approached by the attendants responsible and suborned to give assurance that they had in fact been visited during the times at which the burglaries occurred. Not only the defectives but the men in whose charge they had been supposed to be, were unaware of the absurdity of this alibi. An unfortunate dance-band leader was later found to be the owner of a dress suit found burning in the incinerator.

Much has been written to show both that the defective is and is not prone to sexual

---

* [R. J. A. Berry, R. G. Gordon, *The Mental Defective - a Problem in Social Inefficiency.* London: Kegan Paul, French, Trubner and Co. Ltd., 1931 - Prof. Berry was medical director at Stoke Park]

offences. The imbecile seldom is interested in, or empowered for, a normal heterosexual adventure. The feeble-minded man is generally normal physiologically, he lacks control of his impulses and lacks moral self-judgement. Obviously therefore he is a frequent source of sexual misdemeanours. In Colony life, comparative segregation of course occurs, heterosexual contacts are few, and when they occur on parole, for example, are usually controlled by fear and lack of invitation. The erotic lustfulness of the male animal is therefore more likely to be directed towards homosexual interferences, or masturbation combined with phantasy. In the first case, friendships between the older higher grade and the younger and lower grade should be broken up at once by as great a degree of separation as the Colony will allow. In the second case, much erotic phantasy can be avoided by censoring illustrated periodicals and disallowing certain films. I doubt if the passive agent or receptor type of homosexual exists to any special extent among defectives. Where it occurs, more imbecility per se is the simple and probably correct explanation. Mutual masturbation also occurs between patients at this level, and is most often simply an act of mechanical relief, though the high-grade lascivious defective may so debauch a young imbecile lad as his idea of fun. Such patients should be segregated among their own grade and kind if at all possible. Perhaps some day they may qualify for acceptance to a State Institution [such as Rampton], for I think they can reasonably be called dangerous.

Absconding is another great problem for the Colony which is not enclosed, more particularly just now with grossly inadequate staffing. The delinquent type is naturally more prone to make the attempts, and those known to do so should be kept under day and night supervision, for convenience in a party, under a carefully selected male nurse. It is quite common for this procedure alone to cure the habit and eventually induce sincere co-operation. For one thing it is found that they "lose face" with the more orderly and quiet living higher grade men whose opinions matter. They learn also that not until co-operation is offered genuinely and supported by good conduct, can they hope to get one of the plum occupations.

Our patients of this class only differ from many in the State Institutions in that they are not labelled violent or dangerous. Such a label cannot be attached in potential, but only after the commission of violence.

Such is the seamy side. My reason for stressing it is to support the plea that a Colony whose circumstances cause it to be populated with a higher proportion of delinquent defectives, (whose natural bias is to be troublesome and hard to manage) should be staffed with reliable well-disciplined men in greater numbers proportionate to patients than that accepted in the general deficiency Colony. Some architectural protection against truancy Is also necessary as we have found during the war years. Segregation of the hard cases, failures and debauchers in a special section so that their misdeeds do not disturb the Colony as a whole is probably also necessary. At the present time of course these proposals are like crying for the moon. Men suitable for the care of defectives are not found among the constitutional or professional misfits which is all the Ministry of Labour Offices can offer. And the time for replanning and rebuilding is not quite yet.

I have on a previous occasion expressed the view that in this class of mental deficiency work there need not be a prodigality of certificated male nurses. The new Rushcliffe grade of "nursing assistant" fully meets my idea that suitable sound minded men who may not have the examination gift, can yet handle our patients successfully. A small nucleus of certificated male nurses is sufficient, I feel sure. A high proportion of craftsmen is worth while in the other ranks.

It has been found at Brentry that far from all delinquent defectives of higher grades can be roused to interest in agricultural work. Most such jobs are too tedious and strenuous, for this is a lazy type unless interest is aroused. The refractory party regard their field labours as punishment. Interest and keenness can best be aroused by a job that gives quick obvious results, even some degree of planning and precision. Jobs that lend distinction to the holder and pander to his vanity are popular. It is well to make use of this factor. Vanity can be converted into self-respect.

Were it not for the possibility of wanton or accidental damage to valuable equipment, machinery and tools, the higher grades, whether delinquent or not, could be wholly employed with instruction and future prospects on the various technical jobs of maintenance. In the years immediately ahead building operations should offer great prospects. A great deal of risk has to betaken in any case just now. One cannot lightly place dangerous tools in their hands yet such trades as the shoe-makers shop produce excellent stabilisation through interest and pride in work. The magnificent craft and trade workshops of the State Institutions must ever be a source of envy to those who lack them.   But do not encourage the patient with a future of normal employment to become a show piece as a skilled rug-maker, basket worker or raffia weaver.

Such occupations are for those whose careers are predestined to be worked out in the Colony.

It is quite certain that an acceptable degree of social stabilisation is possible even from the adult higher grade delinquent defective about whom Dr. Benjacer seemed a trifle too gloomy. Of 70 delinquent defectives admitted since January 1940, 18 have been in the Colony for 12 months or less, 6 are in regular employment on license, 7 are at Agricultural hostels, 5 proceed from the Colony to daily outside employment and 22 are employed in essential Colony duties for which in many cases paid employees would otherwise be necessary. Some authorities connected with licensing or boarding out organisations have stressed that only the high grade imbecile or low grade feeble-minded defective is reliable on license. The higher grade type, however stabilised, can recognise exploitation which it is not possible for the imbecile to do. This may account for some of the keenness of professional foster parents to have "manageable" types. The tendency shown recently to put the defective on license on a properly regulated wage footing is in this connection very welcome.

I must apologise for this rather lengthy paper in a discussion which was to be informed and brief and thank you for your attention.

J. Johnston Mason
Medical Superintendent
Brentry Colony.

Appendix 6 – Staff of the Institution

This is a very imperfect list, gleaned from all the sources that can be mustered. The list is most imperfect for more junior staff and for the period after 1948 it is embarrassing in its omissions. However it was felt that any list, however imperfect, was better than none.

Brentry Consortium 1899 - 1948

Chairmen

Captain Belfield	1899 - 1902
Sir Henry Mather Jackson	1902 - 1904
Canon Parker	1904 - 1908
Sir Henry Mather Jackson	1908 - 1937
Mr W Owen	1937 - 1940
Mr G Gibbs	1940 - 1948

Superintendents and Medical Superintendents.

Rev Harold Nelson Burden:	1899 - 1903 Warden
David Fleck	1903 - 1909 Superintendent and Medical Officer
Commander J Richard Lay R.N.	1909 - 1919 Superintendent
Mr Thomas Lambert	1919 - 1929 Superintendent
Dr R Fitzroy Jarrett	1929 - 1931 Medical Superintendent
Dr G R A de Montjoie Rudolf	1931 - 1936 Medical Superintendent (Visiting role from 1936 and in 1955)
Dr James Johnston Mason	1936 - Medical Superintendent

Doctors:

Dr Omerod	1899 - 1903 Medical Officer
	1903 - 1909 Consulting Medical Officer
	1909 - 1929 Medical Officer

Matrons and Chief Nurses

Mrs Katherine Burden	1899 - 1903 Lady Superintendent
Miss Cottle	1903 - 1908 Matron
Miss Batchelor	1908 - ? Matron
Mrs Lambert	1918 - 1929 Matron
Mr W T Williams	1936 Head Nurse
Mr E C Urch	1936 - 1939 Head Nurse
Mr L Browne	1939 - Head Nurse
Mr Gass	Head Male Attendant in March 1943

Hortham-Brentry Hospital Group Management Committee 1948 - 1974

Chairmen:

Prof. J A Nixon	1948 - 1951
Mr R C L Fuller	1951 - 1952 (Acting Chairman)
Mr F G Jennison	1952 - 1964
Mrs L E Anderson	1964 - 1974

Group Medical Superintendents.

Dr J F Lyons	1948 - 1955
Dr W L Walker	1955 - 1966 (was Senior Registrar in Child Psychiatry on appointment)
Dr J B Gordon-Russell	1967 -

Doctors

Dr A Heaton-Ward	1950 - 1954 Assistant Medical Superintendent
Dr T C Leahy	1955 - ? Senior Hospital Medical Officer
Dr J. Jancar	1962 - 1967 Part time Consultant Psychiatrist (with Stoke Park)
Dr E S Lower	1967 - 1974 Consultant Psychiatrist
Dr A C Fairburn	1965 - 1974 Consultant Psychiatrist (beds almost all at Hortham)
Dr M C C Bird	1971 - 1974 Consultant Psychiatrist

Chief Nurses, Matrons and Managers

Mr S H Dagger	Chief Male Nurse Brentry in 1951 & 55
Mr C H Hallas	Chief Male Nurse in 1962
Mr D E Gilbert	1965 – 1974 Chief Male Nurse Brentry 1965
Mr R W G Howse	1954 - 1974 Group Secretary

Southmead 1974 - 1992

Chairmen:

Managers and Nurses

Mr D E Gilbert	1974 – 1977/8	Chief Male Nurse/
Mr Joseph Archer	1975 - ?	Health District Area Administrator
Ian Semple	1977/8-	District Nursing Officer
Denise Thonson	1980	Senior Nursing Officer
Rosemary Grant	- c1984	Mental Handicap Unit Manager
Alan Carpenter	1984 – 1986	Hospital Manager and
	1986 – 1991	Mental Handicap Unit Manager

Doctors

Dr M C Bird	1974 – 1978 Consultant Psychiatrist
Dr J B Gordon Russell	1974 – 1982 Consultant Psychiatrist
Dr E S Lower	1974 - 1985 Consultant Psychiatrist
Dr A C Fairburn	1974 – 1988 Consultant Psychiatrist
Dr O K Ockelford	1979 – 1981 Consultant Psychiatrist
Dr Sylvia Lewis/Carpenter	1983 – 1992 Consultant Psychiatrist

Dr S. Jayewardene   1985 - 1992 Consultant Psychiatrist

Phoenix NHS Trust 1992 - 2000
Chairmen:

    Mr Derek Smith   1991 - 1997

    Mr Arthur Keefe   1997 - 2000

Managers of Brentry:

Mrs Celia Powell	1991- 1993	Area manager
Peter Conners	1991 - 2	Hospital Manager
George Clemow	1992 - 3	Hospital Manager
Wyn Lewis	1993 -	Assistant Director of Hospitals
Vin Puttay	1993 – 4	Nurse Manager
Brian Currie	1994 – 1999	Nurse Manager
Kris Kistnen	1999 – 2000	Assistant Nurse Manager (acting as Nurse Manager)

Doctors

Dr S. Jayewardene	1992 - 1996	Consultant Psychiatrist (and Medical Director, and Consultant Psychiatrist for Clevedon and Thornbury CLDT's))
Dr Sylvia Carpenter	1992 - 1996	Consultant Psychiatrist (after 1996 Medical Director and Consultant Psychiatrist for Bristol North CLDT)
Dr Helen Sharrard	1996 – 2000	Consultant Psychiatrist for Brentry and Consultant Psychiatrist for Thornbury CLDT.
Dr Joanne Thorpe	1998 – 2000	Clinical Assistant
Dr John Harrison	1992 – 2000	Clinical Assistant
Dr Peter Clark		Clinical Assistant

Bath and West Community Care Trust 2000
Chairman

Mr B. Goodson

Managers

Steve Knight	Hospital Resettlement Manager
Kris Kistnen	Assistant Nurse Manager

Doctors

Dr Sylvia Carpenter	Consultant Psychiatrist for Bristol North CLDT, based in Phoenix House
Dr H Sharrard	Consultant Psychiatrist for Brentry and Consultant Psychiatrist for Thornbury CLDT.
Dr Joanne Thorpe	Clinical Assistant
Dr John Harrison	Clinical Assistant
Dr Peter Clark	Clinical Assistant

Sources of Illustrations.

2. Brentry House
   2.1. reproduced from Humphrey Repton: *Observations on the Theory and Practice of Landscape Gardening; Including some remarks on Grecian and Gothic Architecture; collected from various Mss. In the possession of different Noblemen and Gentlemen: the whole tending to establish fixed Principles in the respective Arts; with many Plates.* London: J.Taylor, 1803
   2.2. *Ibid.*
   2.3. From Peacock's Polite Repository (Dec 1803) - proof at V&A Prints and Drawings Dept Ref: E6753-59-1903. – reproduced with permission.
   2.4. From photograph taken by author September 2001
   2.5. From photograph taken March 2000 by author
   2.6. From postcard 27144 by Aerofilms, taken 14 September 1954, copy at BRO.
   2.7. From drawing by Loxton in Bristol Reference Library (ref: L893). Reproduced with the kind permission of the Bristol Reference Library.
   2.8. From photograph taken March 2000 by author
   2.9. Bristol Reference Library. This is illustrated in Reece Winston Bristol in the 1850s. Second edition (Bristol: Winston, 1978) photo 85. Reproduced with the kind permission of the Bristol Reference Library, from reproduction by Reece Winston Archive and Publishing.
   2.10. From 1882 Ordnance Survey 1:2500 map of Gloucestershire (sheet Gloucestershire LXXI.4]
   2.11. From photograph of unknown date found at Brentry, now at BRO. From the quality of photograph and size of trees it is assumed to be about 1900.

3. The move to an Institution
   3.1. H.N.B.: *Life in Algoma; or, Three Years of a Clergyman's Life and Church Work in that Diocese.* London: S.P.C.K., 1894. Page 146.
   3.2. The National Institutions for Inebriates: *Some particulars of Inebriate Reformatories for Women.* London, 1908. Page 34 (*BRO: 39910/PM/1*)
   3.3. *Ibid.*
   3.4. *Ibid.*
   3.5. From photographs taken March 2000 by author

4. The Royal Victoria Homes (Brentry)
   4.1. Adapted from Ordnance Survey map of 1903.
   4.2. *Forty Views of the Royal Victoria Homes, Brentry, nr Bristol.*1901 (*BRO: 40686/B/BK/1*) page 3.
   4.3. *Ibid.* page 13
   4.4. *Ibid.* page 14
   4.5. *Ibid.* page 22
   4.6. *Ibid.* page 17
   4.7. *Ibid.* page 22
   4.8. *Ibid.* page 6
   4.9. *Ibid.* page 19
   4.10. *Ibid.* page 7
   4.11. *Ibid.* page 15
   4.12. *Ibid.* page 12
   4.13. *Ibid.* page 7
   4.14. *Ibid.* page 11
   4.15. *Ibid.* page 12

5. The Change to Mental Deficiency
   5.1. From *Annual report of the Inspector of Reformatories for 1905.* BPP: 1906[Cd.3246]XVI 1.

5.2. Adapted from plan of drainage system dated 24 October 1922 *BRO:* 40686/B/M/5(m).

5.3. Brentry annual report for 1926 (also in *BRO:* 40686/B/Ph/3)

5.4. Brentry annual report for 1926 (also in *BRO:* 40686/B/Ph/3)

5.5. Brentry annual report for 1926 (also in *BRO:* 40686/B/Ph/3)

5.6. Brentry annual report for 1926 (also in *BRO:* 40686/B/Ph/3)

5.7. Brentry annual report for 1928

5.8. *Bristol Times and Mirror* 12 March 1925. Page 11.

5.9. Brentry annual report for 1928, original photo in private collection.

6. Consolidation

  6.1. Annual report for 1930

  6.2. Annual report for 1931

  6.3. Photograph taken by author March 2000

  6.4. 40686/B/Ph/5 – probably used in annual report for 1935 or 1936

  6.5. Adapted from 1935 Ordnance Survey map

7. The start of the NHS

  7.1. From Brentry Scrap Book (*BRO:* 40686/B/SD/2)

  7.2. From Brentry Scrap Book (*BRO:* 40686/B/SD/2)

  7.3. Photograph taken by Aerofilm – R27144.

  7.4. From Brentry Scrap Book (*BRO:* 40686/B/SD/2)

  7.5. From private collection of band leader, J Phillips.

  7.6. From Brentry Scrap Book (*BRO:* 40686/B/SD/2)

  7.7. From Brentry Scrap Book (*BRO:* 40686/B/SD/2)

  7.8. From Brentry Scrap Book (*BRO:* 40686/B/SD/2)

  7.9. From Brentry Scrap Book (*BRO:* 40686/B/SD/2)

  7.10.   Private collection

8. The 1959 Mental Health Act

  8.1. Private collection of J Phillips.

  8.2. Private collection

  8.3. From Brentry Scrap Book (*BRO:* 40686/B/SD/2)

  8.4. From Brentry Scrap Book (*BRO:* 40686/B/SD/2)

  8.5. Private collection

9. 1969 and its aftermath

  9.1. from collection of photographs on adventure playground – due to be deposited at BRO

10. Southmead Health Authority

  10.1.   From collection of West Air Photography, Weston-super-mare (BZ1865/9), reproduced with permission.

  10.2.   from collection of photographs on adventure playground – due to be deposited at BRO

  10.3.   *Ibid.*

  10.4.   *Ibid.*

11. Phoenix NHS Trust

  11.1.   Photograph taken by author.

  11.2.   *Ibid*

  11.3.   *Ibid*

  11.4.   *Ibid*

  11.5.   *Ibid* - taken 14 October 2000.

12. Epilogue

  12.1.   From 'Master Plan and Design Statement for Brentry House and Park'

Index